Praise for *Staff Educator's Guide to Clinical Orientation*

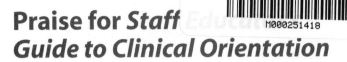

"This is a must-read for educators who develop orientation programs for nurses and for managers, administrators, and others who work with nurses during orientation. Even if you are not involved in orientation, the book provides valuable guidelines for working with nurses who are new to the setting."

–Marilyn H. Oermann, PhD, RN, ANEF, FAAN
Professor and Director of Evaluation and Educational Research
Duke University School of Nursing

"This book shares the hard-earned knowledge acquired through hands-on experience, sweat equity, and application of scholarly rigor. I further applaud the authors for using gender-neutral language as an intentional gesture that promotes a more inclusive reading, education, orientation, and work environment."

–William T. Lecher, MS, MBA, RN, NE-BC
Senior Clinical Director, Cincinnati Children's Hospital Medical Center
President, American Assembly for Men in Nursing

"Jeffery and Jarvis' *Staff Educator's Guide to Clinical Orientation* is a comprehensive and innovative guide to a variety of real-life clinical experiences. This text will be an asset to any nurse educator's collection."

–Cynthia L. Balevre, MSNEd, RN-BC
Nursing Consultant and Educator
Clinical Policy Reviewer, United General Health
Adjunct Nurse Professor, Chamberlain College of Nursing
Assistant Nurse Professor, Colorado Technical University

Staff Educator's Guide to Clinical Orientation

Onboarding Solutions for Nurses

Alvin D. Jeffery, MSN, RN-BC, CCRN, FNP-BC
Robin L. Jarvis, MS, SPHR

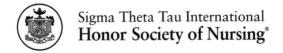

Sigma Theta Tau International
Honor Society of Nursing®

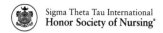

Sigma Theta Tau International
Honor Society of Nursing®

The Honor Society of Nursing, Sigma Theta Tau International (STTI) is a nonprofit organization whose mission is to support the learning, knowledge, and professional development of nurses committed to making a difference in health worldwide. Founded in 1922, STTI has 130,000 members in 86 countries. Members include practicing nurses, instructors, researchers, policymakers, entrepreneurs and others. STTI's 493 chapters are located at 673 institutions of higher education throughout Australia, Botswana, Brazil, Canada, Colombia, Ghana, Hong Kong, Japan, Kenya, Malawi, Mexico, the Netherlands, Pakistan, Portugal, Singapore, South Africa, South Korea, Swaziland, Sweden, Taiwan, Tanzania, United Kingdom, United States, and Wales. More information about STTI can be found online at www.nursingsociety.org.

Sigma Theta Tau International
550 West North Street
Indianapolis, IN, USA 46202

To order additional books, buy in bulk, or order for corporate use, contact Nursing Knowledge International at 888.NKI.4YOU (888.654.4968/US and Canada) or +1.317.634.8171 (outside US and Canada).

To request a review copy for course adoption, email solutions@nursingknowledge.org or call 888. NKI.4YOU (888.654.4968/US and Canada) or +1.317.634.8171 (outside US and Canada).

To request author information, or for speaker or other media requests, contact Marketing, Honor Society of Nursing, Sigma Theta Tau International at 888.634.7575 (US and Canada) or +1.317.634.8171 (outside US and Canada).

ISBN: 9781938835384
EPUB ISBN: 9781938835391
PDF ISBN: 9781938835407
MOBI ISBN: 9781938835414

Library of Congress Cataloging-in-Publication Data

Jeffery, Alvin D., 1986- author.
  Staff educator's guide to clinical orientation : onboarding solutions for nurses / Alvin D. Jeffery, Robin L. Jarvis.
      p. ; cm.
  Includes bibliographical references.
  ISBN 978-1-938835-38-4 (book : alk. paper) -- ISBN 978-1-938835-39-1 (EPUB) -- ISBN 978-1-938835-40-7 (PDF) -- ISBN 978-1-938835-41-4 (MOBI)
  I. Jarvis, Robin L., 1962- author. II. Sigma Theta Tau International, issuing body. III. Title.
  [DNLM: 1. Inservice Training--methods. 2. Nurses. 3. Inservice Training--organization & administration. 4. Professional Competence. WY 18.5]
  RT76
  610.73071'55--dc23

First Printing, 2014

Publisher: Renee Wilmeth
Acquisitions Editor: Emily Hatch
Editorial Coordinator: Paula Jeffers
Cover Designer: Michael Tanamachi
Interior Design/Page Layout: Katy Bodenmiller

Principal Book Editor: Carla Hall
Development and Project Editor: Kevin Kent
Copy Editor: Erin Geile
Proofreader: Barbara Bennett
Indexer: Jane Palmer

Dedication

We would like to dedicate this to our partners, Jamey Rutschilling and Susan Brodeur, for their love and support for us during the writing of this book and our respective journeys. Also, we dedicate this book in memory of our grandfather and father, Kenneth D. Jarvis, who taught both of us that if you could read about it, you could do something about it.

Acknowledgments

We would like to acknowledge the following people for their willingness to review and offer feedback on the content of this book:

David D. Jarvis, for providing insights from the perspective of nursing home facilities, for making sure that things made sense, and for being a great uncle and brother!

Bill Jeffery, for offering guidance on the flow of content, for providing some humorous remarks, and for being a great nephew and brother!

Dena Clark and Beth Mueller, for making sure Alvin stayed on topic but also included all the important information for educators. Dena and Beth are two of the most remarkable nurse educators, colleagues, and friends, and Alvin loved every day he was able to work with them.

Robin would like to acknowledge Debra R. France, EdD, who, with Robin, codesigned and developed SEMATECH's orientation program. Debra is a gifted learning and development professional and someone to whom Robin always will look for ideas, camaraderie, and creativity.

About the Authors

Alvin D. Jeffery, MSN, RN-BC, CCRN, FNP-BC

Alvin D. Jeffery is currently a full-time PhD student at Vanderbilt University in Nashville, Tennessee. He holds part-time appointments as an education consultant at Cincinnati Children's Hospital Medical Center in Cincinnati, Ohio, and as an adjunct instructor with several colleges and universities.

Jeffery's most recent full-time job was working as the unit-based educator in a pediatric intensive care unit at Cincinnati Children's Hospital Medical Center. During this time as an educator, Jeffery finished his master of science in nursing (MSN) degree with a focus as a family nurse practitioner (FNP). He is board-certified in both Nursing Professional Development (American Nurses Credentialing Center) and Pediatric Critical-Care Nursing (American Association of Critical-Care Nurses), and he has developed and instructed internal review courses for both of these certifications.

Jeffery has facilitated several internal in-services/continuing education programs in various aspects of nursing professional and staff development and has served as a preceptor for several new educators in the pediatric intensive care unit. He has collaborated with almost every department in the organization, design, and development of various staff development projects including, but not limited to, competency assessment tools, education record management databases, simulation implementation, and preceptor development.

Robin L. Jarvis, MS, SPHR

Robin L. Jarvis is an expert in adult learning with more than 20 years of experience in high technology, retail, and consulting companies. She has experience in leadership development and other interpersonal training as well as serving as an HR generalist and leading a talent acquisition team. Her work has taken her from Texas to India, China, Singapore, Taiwan, and England.

In addition to a master of science in leadership, Jarvis has participated in more than 500 hours of additional training in topics such as cross-cultural communication, accelerated learning, instructional design, leadership development, and facilitation. She has designed and delivered workshops on topics including new employee orientation and onboarding, change management, employee engagement, career development, accelerated learning, learning styles, Myers-Briggs Type Indicator (MBTI), StrengthsFinder, *The Seven Habits of Highly Effective People,* presentation skills, meeting skills, behavioral-based interviewing and many other topics.

Jarvis has copresented at International Society for Performance Improvement (ISPI) conferences on the topic of orientation and onboarding. She and Debra R. France, EdD, co-authored an article, "Quick Starts for New Employees," which was published in *Training and Development* magazine. She and France received SEMATECH's corporate award for the orientation program they designed.

Table of Contents

Foreword

There is nothing that can start a new job better than a great orientation experience, and there is nothing that can make you question your decision to join an organization more than a bad orientation experience. For an organization, orientation can be opportunity seized or opportunity wasted.

Transitions are critical times, whether the transition is to a new organization, a new specialty, or a new role. Never are you more excited in your career or more vulnerable than when you are in transition. Even nurses who were considered experts in their last position or role are vulnerable when they start a job at a new organization or move into a new role or specialty. For new employees, how they are welcomed, communicated with, and supported in orientation sets the tone for the entire time they are with the organization. If the new employees are also new graduates, orientation also influences and serves as a critical part of the foundation for their entire careers. How organizations facilitate these transitions has long-term effects on the success of the nurse as an individual and the organization as a whole.

Marilyn Ferguson, an American futurist, in describing transitions, says, "It's not so much that we're afraid of change or so in love with the old ways, but it's that place in between that we fear…It's like being between trapezes. It's Linus when his blanket is in the dryer. There's nothing to hold on to." Staff educators create safe environments for transition and are the bridge between the old world and the new. They help orientees understand and ultimately meet the clinical and cultural expectations of their new world.

Unfortunately, orientation is too often taken for granted and is seen as something that must be endured, rather than appreciated as the front line of defense for safe patient care and one of the best risk management tools available to the organization. Orientation done well assures the competence of orientees and builds the confidence they need to practice their profession.

Staff education is a specialty all its own. It requires a set of knowledge and expertise above and beyond what is required to be a good clinical nurse. Staff educators must be knowledgeable, flexible, and nimble. Providing orientation in a clinical environment demands the ability not only to teach in a planned way, but also to recognize and take advantage of teachable moments as they present themselves. Orientation is rarely, if ever, a one-size-fits-all proposition. Though the ultimate required knowledge and competencies may be the same, the orientees are not. Successful orientation for a new graduate nurse requires a very different path than orientation for an experienced critical-care nurse.

In this book, Alvin D. Jeffery and Robin L. Jarvis provide a resource to help staff educators make orientation successful for the orientees and the organization. With a pragmatic, reality-based approach, they offer guidance on all aspects of providing an effective clinical orientation. Jeffery and Jarvis know that orientation does not exist in isolation and that stakeholders must be consulted to understand their expectations of orientation and to provide feedback on its effectiveness. They also know that in the real world, problems occur—instructional technology doesn't work, an emergency puts the orientation plans on hold, a preceptor-preceptee relationship just isn't working, or an orientee is in distress—and they provide information and thoughtful suggestions on ways to solve those problems. They also offer valuable resources including worksheets, tools, how-to-do-it hints, and even a chapter on practical steps for organizing the complex work and information required for orientation.

This book has the potential to influence the careers of many nurses and positively impact patient care. Think of the hundreds of nurse orientees each staff educator influences. Then think of the thousands of patients each of those nurse orientees will care for throughout their careers. Now you begin to understand the importance and value of supporting staff educators and providing them with resources such as this book that help them create, provide, evaluate, and improve orientations.

–Beth Ulrich, EdD, RN, FACHE, FAAN
Senior Partner, Innovative Health Resources
Editor, Nephrology Nursing Journal
Author, Mastering Precepting: A Nurse's Handbook for Success

Introduction

"I never teach my pupils; I only attempt to provide the conditions in which they can learn." –Albert Einstein

Welcome to the *Staff Educator's Guide to Clinical Orientation*! Throughout this book, we want to provide you with tools and techniques for creating and sustaining those ideal conditions to which Einstein refers. We hope you'll find this book an enjoyable and insightful discussion of how to develop orientation and onboarding programs for nurses that will result in well-prepared orientees and satisfied organizational stakeholders.

Our goal in writing this book is to provide you with a quick reference or just-in-time field guide to making your orientation programs successful. We know that you have a busy schedule, so we have included several worksheets and tools that can be used immediately in case you don't have the time to read a more lengthy discussion on a particular topic. We hope you eventually will get time to read the entire book so that you can understand the tools and adapt them more to your individual needs, but we wanted to give you something you could use today.

We have written this text for nursing professional development specialists (that is, nurse educators in the clinical setting) as well as managers and administrators who work with nurses in orientation. Although preceptors and senior-level administrators may learn new concepts from these readings, the intended audience includes those mid-level leaders who dabble in day-to-day orientation/onboarding activities as well as the design, development, and implementation of orientation/onboarding programs. Our experience has shown that many mid-level leaders are not fully equipped in formal training and development concepts that are essential to effective and efficient orientation/onboarding programs. This book is intended to help bridge this knowledge gap.

Because we want you to use this as a field guide, we are providing an overview of each chapter so that you know right where to go for your specific issue or concern. Each chapter has some suggested reflection/discussion questions for you to consider. We hope that you find these questions, as well as the worksheets, tables, etc., helpful.

Chapter 1—"Important Considerations for Onboarding and Orientation": This chapter provides you with an overview of the ADDIE model (Analyze, Design, Develop, Implement, and Evaluate), which is the standard model for designing training programs such as onboarding and orientation. You might notice the similarities between the ADDIE model and one you use every day in nursing (Assess, Diagnose, Plan, Implement, and Evaluate).

The ADDIE model really provides the basis for the rest of the book. We look at each step in the model throughout the book. The remainder of Chapter 1 looks at *principles* and *principals* for your program. Principles are key things to consider during the development of your program. The principals are all the stakeholders in this important program and process.

Chapter 2—"Analyzing and Designing an Orientation Program": Chapter 2 looks at the first two steps in the ADDIE model—Analyze and Design. In the Analyze step, we address a few data gathering modes and even provide a focus group agenda for you to use. If you have an existing program, we provide some tips on how to assess the strengths and weaknesses of your program, as well as provide some errors to avoid. If you're creating a new program, this chapter will give you the tools you need to get started by ensuring you know what the needs of the organization are.

During the Analyze step, you must understand your learners, so we talk about some models that address how people learn. We limit it to three models, as we believe that the application of these three will ensure that your learners' needs are met. Many of you are familiar with the American Association of Critical-Care Nurses' (AACN) Synergy Model, and we discuss how that can be applied to your analysis and design. We also discuss making recommendations to key stakeholders when you have finished the Analyze phase, and we provide some worksheets and examples to get you started with the Design phase.

Chapter 3—"Developing and Implementing an Orientation Program": This chapter takes the design worksheets we introduced in Chapter 2 and guides you on how to use those to develop your orientation and onboarding modules. We provide examples at the organizational and unit level, just as we did in Chapter 2. We also include examples of facilitator notes and pages from Participant Guides.

In Chapter 3, we address the concepts of centralized and decentralized programs. These concepts are especially important for those of you working in larger organizations; however, regardless of the size of your organization, you should be addressing items at the organization and unit levels. We also take a peek at a unit's onboarding program and, specifically, the importance of the preceptor.

Chapter 4—"Evaluating an Individual's Competency": This chapter may be the most important chapter in the book because at the end of the day your onboarding and orientation program should ensure that each new nurse is working in a safe and competent manner. The first thing we address is whether time-based or competency-based programs are more effective. We believe that competency-based is best; however, we also are well aware of organizational challenges, such as budgeting, scheduling, etc.

The remainder of the chapter is devoted to competence—what it is, what it isn't, how to evaluate it, and what to do if you are not seeing it. We make some distinctions between competence and confidence that we know you will find useful. Additionally, we delineate between cognitive learning, psychomotor skills, and affective thoughts and behaviors and provide some tips on how to teach each and how to evaluate each.

Chapter 5—"Working With Orientees": Okay, maybe this is the most important chapter! In this chapter, we identify several different types of orientees:

- The new college graduate
- The experienced nurse
- The nurse who is progressing quickly
- The one who has made an error
- The one who doesn't get along with his/her preceptor
- The one who has a learning style that is different from his/her preceptor
- The one who struggles with interpersonal communication
- The one who wants to quit
- The one who likely will not complete onboarding successfully

Whew! This chapter provides specific examples of what an orientee may do or experience and provides practical tips for what a preceptor and/or nurse educator can do to help the orientee be successful.

Chapter 6—"Evaluating an Orientation Program": Chapter 6 looks at different models of evaluation. You will note some overlap of the models, and that is on purpose. The bottom line with evaluation is that (a) you must be able to show that the orientees are successful after completing the program and (b) the principal stakeholders can see that the program is efficient and cost-effective.

We provide examples of evaluation at the organization and unit levels to help you as you navigate the evaluation process. A key point in evaluation is that you must begin thinking about it during the Analysis phase, as Analysis is where you determine what you want people to be able to do better and/or differently as a result of your program.

Chapter 7—"Regulatory Considerations": We would be remiss if we didn't include information for you about accreditation bodies, federal regulations, and the like. This chapter highlights the importance of working with your Human Resources professionals as well as key pieces of legislation that may impact you and your orientees. We also discuss the importance of documentation and talk about when, where, and how long to document it and keep it.

Chapter 8—"Practical Steps for Staying Organized": Juggling orientees, paperwork, and schedules can be overwhelming. In our final chapter, we provide easy-to-implement ideas for keeping your electronic and paper files organized. We also discuss ways to use email and calendar software to keep the schedule from getting the best of you.

We have also provided an appendix that lists some of our favorite books, websites, literature, etc., regarding onboarding and orientation. We hope that you find the book helpful, enlightening, and perhaps even a bit humorous from time to time.

As you can see from what we plan on covering in each chapter, we aim to provide a well-rounded approach to creating and sustaining high-quality orientation and onboarding programs that meet the needs of the individual, the organization, and the patients they serve. By providing you with a combination of practical advice and theoretically sound recommendations, we intend for you to have everything you need at your fingertips to ensure a successful orientation and onboarding program.

Whether you're new to leading orientation efforts or a seasoned nursing staff development specialist, we think you will find this book a great addition to your personal library. Once you've finished reading it, we hope you'll have new perspectives, found a greater insight, or at least gained a few nuggets of how to do some things better. Regardless of what you discover along the way, we hope you enjoy the journey through these pages as much as we enjoy sharing them with you!

CHAPTER 1

Important Considerations for Onboarding and Orientation

Introduction

Hiring someone takes time, money, and your energy! You spend time:

- Making sure the job description is up-to-date
- Reviewing resumes
- Conducting telephone interviews
- Deciding whom to bring to your organization for interviews
- Interviewing and observing the candidate in your "natural habitat"
- Deciding which candidate is the best fit for your unit, your team, and your organization

Whew! That *is* a lot of time and energy. So, now that the new person is starting, do you leave his or her success to chance? Really?!?! As Dr. Phil would say, "How's that working for ya?"

You would not have picked up this book if you didn't realize that there's something missing in the way you bring new nurses to your organization. Studies suggest that organizations retain new employees longer and those employees are more successful when they have experienced orientation and onboarding. According to a white paper written by David Freeman (2013):

- Up to 4% of new employees will quit after the first day.

- Most employees make up their minds within the first 6 months if they want to stay with the organization.

- 22% of new employee turnover occurs within the first 45 days.

- Hiring costs are now estimated to be three times the employee's annual salary.

- With a good onboarding process, 58% of your employees can still be with you 3 years later.

You may be wondering what the difference is between onboarding and orientation. Technically, *orientation* is an event—from a half-day "here is the cafeteria" to a multiday workshop. On the other hand, *onboarding* is a process that really starts the day the candidate accepts the job offer. We will talk about both the event and the process throughout this book, and we will refer to both terms somewhat interchangeably. Both play important roles in ensuring that your new hire is successful and stays with your organization. Laurano (2013) notes that "only 37% of organizations have invested in strategic onboarding for longer than two years" (p. 5). That means that about two-thirds of organizations are doing little or nothing to help their new employees be successful and/or to welcome them to the organization.

Pause for a moment and consider your first day on the job...or even your first day as a new nurse. You may have to reach back quite a way to rediscover those thoughts and feelings (especially if they were so traumatic that you *tried* to forget them). We bet the emotions you experienced then aren't too different from what new employees in your organization are going to experience. Therefore, use your own memories to set the stage or context for the journey on which your new employees are about to embark. We want to help *you* help *them* in making this one of the greatest journeys in which they will ever participate.

We do want to highlight what we think works well and how you can integrate it into your organization. Let's contrast two different onboarding experiences to bring some of the things that work well to light.

ONBOARD OR OVERBOARD?

To help illustrate the differences between a "good" or "bad" initial experience (or if you want a little reminder of what starting as a new nurse might feel like), check out the stories of Nate and Ron, who started as new graduate nurses in two very different environments. Nate had a positive experience that contributed to his professional success and was effectively onboarded. In contrast, Ron received a less than ideal introduction to his organization and was, shall we say, overboarded.

Nate started as a float pool nurse at a large urban hospital. While he was initially frustrated by a lengthy organizational orientation before starting to work with patients, he was well-equipped with in-depth knowledge of the organization's mission, vision, values, policies, procedures, and processes. Once he was able to begin working with patients, he not only had an assigned manager, educator, and preceptor, but he also was immediately matched with a mentor who checked in frequently on his progress. Being a float pool nurse, Nate did not spend more than 2–4 weeks on one unit, which could have easily led to the inability to develop meaningful relationships with his colleagues. However, the structured assignment of key personnel and frequently scheduled progress meetings ensured Nate felt connected and cared for. He was also invited to social events occurring offsite, which assisted with his learning informal culture. Multiple education modules and classes, while a seemingly impossible task at first, occurred throughout his orientation experience, and by the 6-month mark, he was not only knowledgeable of appropriate practices but also began teaching newer nurses. Nate was successfully onboarded and quickly became a leader in the organization.

Ron started as an emergency department nurse in a small rural hospital. Due to a staffing crisis in the department, the manager did not allow new employees to attend formal organizational orientation. Instead, Ron had to watch videos of recorded orientation sessions in his spare time to

continues

*learn about the organization's mission, vision, and values. Initially, Ron
was quite excited that he was able to care for patients on his first day at
work. However, the excitement he experienced during the first few days
quickly faded because he did not have a consistent preceptor or mentor
to assess his progress. No one was able to provide Ron with feedback,
and he discovered that practices varied widely between nurses. A lack
of classes and education modules meant Ron had to spend time off the
clock looking for information from his nursing school textbooks. After
3 weeks, Ron's manager did a "drive by" meeting where she asked Ron if
he would be fine without a designated preceptor starting the next day.
Not feeling comfortable enough to verbalize his uneasiness, he complied.
Then 6 weeks later, Ron was working large amounts of overtime, had
no meaningful peer relationships, and unknowingly performed many
procedures incorrectly. Unfortunately, one of these procedures resulted
in the death of a patient, and he decided not to return to work. Ron was
overboarded, and he moved out of state to find a new job.*

*While the negative example might seem a little extreme, we do hope it
illustrates the impact that even small negative experiences can have on
a new employee. This book is devoted to helping you with every aspect
of your orientation program and hopefully turning your overboarding
nightmares into onboarding successes.*

The ADDIE Model

So, how do we get started on this journey of creating great programs?
Luckily for nurses, there's a systematic approach to instructional design
that is almost identical to the nursing process (you remember Assess,
Diagnose, Plan, Implement, and Evaluate, right?). In instructional
design, this process is called the ADDIE model (Figure 1.1). ADDIE
stands for Analyze, Design, Develop, Implement, and Evaluate
(Branson, et al., 1975). This is a process used by instructional designers
and educators to develop programs that meet the needs of their
respective organizations. For our purposes, it will be used to create and/
or modify an onboarding and orientation program.

NOTE

*If you are looking for more information about ADDIE, check out this
website: http://nwlink.com/~donclark/history_isd/addie.html*

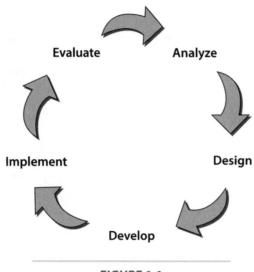

FIGURE 1.1

The ADDIE model for instructional design.

Analyze

In Analyze, it is important to ask the right questions. In Chapter 2 we go deeper into this phase and discuss how to gather the data needed for an onboarding and orientation program. We will look at some key questions right now. Once the questions are answered, it is time to begin the real analysis. Here are some questions to use as you finish data-gathering and begin to really absorb, sort, and make sense of the data.

- Who are the learners and what are their commonalities and differences?
- What behaviors and skills do you want to see them execute successfully?
- What constraints exist that may prevent them from performing successfully?
- What methods will you employ to help them learn and practice?
- What adult learning theories might you need to apply throughout the program?
- What existing content and/or materials do you have?

- What is your timeline for completion?

Once you have the analysis done, you have a better understanding of the scope of the project. You have your parameters set and can start the next phase in the ADDIE model, Design.

Design

The Design phase is fun! When you think about Design, consider this story. Years ago, a new elementary school was built. School started before the fence could be built around the playground. Before the fence was built, the children stayed close to the school and the playground equipment. After the fence was built, the children played on every single inch of the playground. So, what's the moral of the story? Creativity needs parameters. You already discovered these parameters during the Analysis phase, so your creativity during Design must keep these parameters in mind. Some of them will include:

- **Learning Objectives**—Does the program help the new employees meet the learning objectives of the program?

- **Scalability**—How easily can the program be delivered multiple times with small or large numbers of employees?

- **Pragmatism**—Does the program represent reality for the participants or are we taking them on a sci-fi adventure? Reality is best!

- **Cost**—How much does it cost per person, or per run of the program? Your leader will appreciate it if you can build a "champagne" program on a "beer" budget.

CHAMPAGNE PROGRAMS ON A BEER BUDGET

- **Reach out to other departments.** *Often, the staffing, PR, or Marketing departments will have "freebies" with your organization's logo imprinted. They may share those with you, and your new employees will love having some cool logo stuff!*

- **Reuse content that already exists.** *This saves you time and development dollars.*

- **Small investments can save big dollars.** *For example, buy a digital camcorder. Now, rather than paying for professional videos,* *you can shoot and use your own!*

- **Go low-tech and get creative!** *You don't need a mannequin for practicing dressing changes when paper plates will work.*
- **Become friends with people in Central Supply!** *They often have items that are expiring that you wouldn't use on a patient, but your orientees could practice with those supplies.*

While many of you have looked at scalability, tend to be pragmatic as most good nurses are, and are usually concerned about cost, we are guessing that writing learning objectives may not be something you do regularly or have done...ever. Learning objectives can be an art unto themselves. Here are three guidelines for developing good learning objectives.

1. **Action/task**—A well-written objective includes an action, that is, something that can be observed or heard. For example, "Administer medicine" would be part of a good objective because you can observe the nurse doing just that. "Understand policies" would not be a good objective because you cannot observe whether or not someone understands the policies.

2. **Performance measures**—What are the criteria on which success is based? In the "Administer medicine" example, we might add "within 30 minutes of receiving orders" and "at the correct dosage 100% of the time."

3. **Conditions**—Under what conditions will the action be performed? To complete our example, we might say, "Administer medicine at the correct dosage 100% of the time within 30 minutes of receiving orders during any assigned shift and unit."

CAN YOU FIND THE WELL-WRITTEN OBJECTIVES?

1. *Appreciate classical music by researching and discussing Beethoven's Fifth Symphony.*
2. *Update patient record within 30 minutes of seeing patient 100% of the time.*
3. *Communicate effectively with patient families 100% of the time.*
4. *Know how to deliver IV medication.*

Okay, which ones are well-written? You probably guessed that the first

continues

one is bad. How can you measure someone's appreciation of classical music? You can't! Let's look at the other ones.

Number 2 is well-written. It contains an action, "Update patient record..." a performance measure, "...within 30 minutes of seeing patient..." and the conditions, "...100% of the time."

Number 3 is well-written with the exception of the performance measure. How do we measure effective communication? We need more specificity on that in order to provide feedback.

The final one is bad. We cannot measure "Know," we don't have criteria to determine success, and we don't specify conditions under which the action must be done.

The bottom line about learning objectives? They provide the road map for the Design, Development, Implementation, and Evaluation. If the learning objectives are not met by the participants, the program is unsuccessful...period.

THE ADDIE MODEL IN ACTION

Robin and her colleague, Debra R. France, EdD, were asked to develop an orientation program for a company that had 30-35% annual turnover (by design). The company was a research-and-development consortium that brought together people from 14 different companies. These companies competed with each other in the marketplace, but had to get along in the confines of the consortium. Robin and Debra had a challenging task.

Their analysis concluded that people needed to know what the culture and behavioral expectations were and needed an opportunity to practice them before being turned loose. They developed learning objectives that would meet these culture and behavioral expectations. Additionally, they found that much of the work was done in meetings. To this end, they developed a 3-day workshop called "Beyond Competitive Boundaries" that incorporated meeting skills, team skills, listening skills, and diversity appreciation. By the time they gathered all the content they wanted to use, they had about 10 days of content.

In order to make it work in a 3-day workshop, they got creative. They employed accelerated learning concepts to shorten the time needed to acquire skills. The design included putting participants into mock project teams (low-tech simulation), and as the teams worked through the project, they were given opportunities to practice all the skills needed to be successful at the consortium. At the end of the 3 days, each team had to share with an executive what it had learned about the importance of collaboration in the consortium environment. Teams presented skits, taught the executives to line dance (it was the early 1990s), developed fun flowcharts, and came up with unique ways to share their experience. During the several years that Robin and Debra ran the workshop, they did not ever see the same presentation twice. Robin and Debra received the Corporate Excellence Award for creating the new and improved orientation program.

Additionally, there were 2 days that bookended the workshop. The first day had originally been a "death by PowerPoint" day that they changed significantly. They worked with the presenters (HR, Finance, IT, etc.) to develop creative ways of presenting their information:

- *To learn the building layout, they created a scavenger hunt.*
- *To learn the key HR policies, small groups were assigned different policies and had to teach each other about their respective policies.*
- *To learn about the harassment and discrimination policies, participants were given scenarios and asked to rate them on a scale. An employment law attorney facilitated the discussion.*
- *The last day of the week was devoted to safety training, as the consortium's site contained a clean room environment. The safety training was very hands-on, so it required little rework during the design process. (France & Jarvis, 1996)*

Development

During Development, you start creating supporting materials and resources (paper and/or electronic), finalizing how different sections of the content will be delivered or facilitated, and finalizing the flow of the program. That said, there are some basic things you need to consider during Development that will help you reach learners most effectively.

The first is the concept of flow. Flow means that you must arrange activities, lectures, demonstrations, etc., in a way that keeps the learners engaged and allows for the greatest efficacy. One way to think about it is from the perspectives of the facilitator/instructor and the learner/student (Figure 1.2).

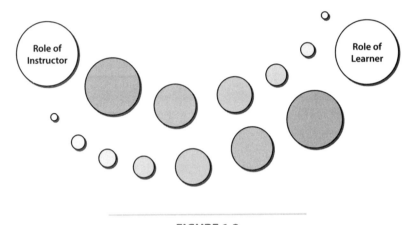

FIGURE 1.2

Role of instructor/role of learner in learning.

We developed this model through informal conversations with students and facilitators of accelerated learning. At the beginning of a learning session, the role of the instructor or facilitator is large, as this is where the instructor explains and/or demonstrates what is to be learned. Note that as the process continues the role of the student or learner becomes more prominent, so that by the end, the facilitator is providing feedback as the student demonstrates the new skill. This concept may be repeated over and over (microlevel) throughout an onboarding program and also at a metalevel as you design the entire program.

During Development, you will want to consider different methods for delivery of the content. These methods may include:

- **Instructor-led**—May be used for group learning or one-on-one learning. Instructor-led modules may include lectures (less than 20 minutes in length), practice opportunities, etc.

- **E-learning**—This method is great for short bursts of information. Ideally, you would not want an e-learning organizational module to be longer than approximately 45 minutes. Longer modules may make it difficult for the learner to stay engaged with the content. At the unit level, clinicians prefer shorter, 10-to-15-minute modules, as those are easier to work into their regular schedules.

- **Job aids**—Provide step-by-step references for specific activities. Often, these are activities that are not completed by someone on a regular basis. An organizational example would be how to complete an expense report, which is something that most clinicians may not do on a regular basis. At the unit level, this could include how to dilute a rarely administered medication or how to document patient information in the electronic medical record. Most job aids are electronic and available via the organization's intranet.

- **Simulations**—Although many people think of simulations as high-tech, it is possible to have low-tech and effective simulations, such as that mentioned earlier in the chapter. Even in nursing, low-tech simulations may be as simple as practicing central venous catheter dressing changes using a paper plate.

Implementation and Evaluation

Implementation is where the rubber meets the road, so to speak. You have done your analysis, developed your learning objectives, and designed and developed a program to meet those objectives. You have created the appropriate materials needed. Now, all you need are your new nurses! For more on developing and implementing an onboarding program, see Chapter 3.

Evaluation is a critical component of the model and should be considered during Analysis and Design, especially. Evaluation should be conducted at the program level and the individual level. See Chapter 6 for more details about evaluation methods and models.

ADDIE is a great model to use as you design your new (or improve your existing) orientation and onboarding program. It provides enough structure to keep you focused on your goal and allows for creativity in the design, development, and implementation of your program. You'll find that this book is laid out in a format similar to the ADDIE model.

Principles and Principals of Onboarding

With all these principles and principals about, you might feel like you're back in school. And, if you have never received formal training in managing orientation or onboarding programs, then to some degree, you are. In this section, we provide you with principles and principals of successful onboarding:

- *Principles* are the guidelines to keep in mind while analyzing, designing, developing, and implementing an onboarding and orientation program.

- *Principals* are the key people who need to be involved in the development, implementation, and sustainability of the program.

Think of the principles as the foundation and framework of a building—if absent, the contents are exposed, unsupported, and likely to collapse. If we go with the same illustration, then the principals are the people who will inhabit, maintain, or provide resources for the building. All of these people will want (and need) to provide input into its construction.

We want to start with the principles of successful onboarding. Although we have divided these important components into three arenas, you will see overlap between them—for example, engagement is part of implementation, but must be considered during design as well.

The key principles of onboarding are:

- Analysis and Design Principles
  - Answer the right questions with your process and program.
  - Be clear about job, team, and organizational responsibilities.
  - Leverage appropriate models.
- Development and Implementation Principles
  - Engage the employees each and every day.
  - Provide (and accept) feedback early and often.

- Evaluation Principles
  - Base the evaluation on the program objectives.
  - Evaluate the participants and the program regularly.

Analysis/Design Principle 1: Answer the Right Questions with Your Process and Program

Many orientation programs start with the premise that people need to know how to efficiently move throughout the building. Yes, they do; however, are those really the most important things they need to know? Probably not. For your program and process to be successful, you need to start with determining the most essential prerequisites for a new employee, and that begins with asking and answering some very important questions.

For example, one question you might want to answer is, "What does it take for someone to be successful in this nursing environment?" This question will lead you to areas of regulations and compliance, as well as understanding the types of patients your organization assists and the organizational culture. To really answer these questions well, you will need to engage with the principals (key stakeholders). We will discuss different ways to engage with the principals later in this chapter.

We have provided several starting questions for you here (Worksheet 1.1), but feel free to modify these or add more of your own. As you are brainstorming which questions to include in your organization, if you find yourself debating whether or not to include a question, we would recommend you do include it here. Once you begin developing and implementing the program's components, it can be very difficult to return to the design stage to make changes should additional information surface later. Asking more questions and gathering more information are best at this point in the game.

WORKSHEET 1.1 *Key Analysis Questions for Onboarding*

QUESTION	ANSWER
What does it take for someone to be successful in this nursing environment?	
How do we know if someone is successful within the first 30, 60, and 90* days?	
Whom do our new nurses need to meet within their first 30, 60, and 90 days?	
What additional skills or knowledge might they need within the first 30, 60, and 90 days?	
What do we already have in place to help them as they join our organization?	

Note: 30, 60, and 90 days are commonly used time frames in Human Resources for performance evaluations, but for training in highly specialized areas (such as an operating room or intensive care unit), longer time frames may be more appropriate.

We want you to look at these questions (from Worksheet 1.1) one by one to understand what type of information is requested.

What does it take for someone to be successful in this nursing environment? To answer this question, you will need a great deal of information about the work at an individual, team, and organizational level. A job description is often a good place to start. The challenge is to dig deeper with that question. Most of us have experienced working somewhere and feeling like we hadn't yet inherited the secret book of knowledge. That feeling has to do with the corporate culture. In *The Corporate Culture Survival Guide*, Edgar H. Schein (2009) notes that there are three levels of culture:

1. **Artifacts**—These are organizational structure and processes that you can see, but you may have a hard time understanding. For example, do people use titles, that is, "Doctor Smith," or do they use first names, and why?

2. **Espoused Values**—These are the things the organization values and talks about. However, the actions of the people within the organization may not always support the espoused values. For example, to what degree should a new hire be able to align his/her personal work with the mission and vision of the organization?

3. **Share Tacit Assumptions**—These are the things that are in that secret book of knowledge we just mentioned. These include things such as knowing that if Joe has shut his car door really firmly, you might want to avoid him for a couple of hours. Or, additionally, learning the financial and budgeting cycle so that you know when to ask to go to the next conference. Those are things that you may assume your new employees know, but they don't…yet.

Now that you've articulated the what, it's time to talk about how you know that someone is successful in this environment. How do you know? You know because the person is meeting and, likely, exceeding the job responsibilities (for additional information on assessing the ability to competently perform job responsibilities, check out Chapter 4). You know because the nurse is interacting in culture-appropriate ways with patients and other staff. You know because Joe slammed the door, and your nurse waited until after lunch to approach him about the nonemergency situation.

Be explicit—very detailed—when answering the first two questions on the worksheet. If you can describe what and how the person needs to do the job effectively, you are well on your way to developing a great onboarding program.

The last three questions on the worksheet provide additional insight and information that you'll need:

- The first has to do with "whom" your nurse needs to meet and when. It is easy to overwhelm a new person with (pardon the expression) "death by introductions." Really take the time to map out whom the new nurse needs to know and when. Start with the key staff in the unit and go from there. This could include fellow nurses, management/leadership, physicians, unlicensed assistive personnel, and ancillary staff (physical/ occupational/speech therapists, respiratory therapists, child life specialists, chaplains, etc.).

- As you think about what additional skills and knowledge the nurse might need, keep pace in mind. The person is not going to be "perfect" on the job the first day…or even the 30th day; however, you can start to identify the additional skills and knowledge the person will need. For example, in an organization where all staff are involved in shared governance, it might be important to have some knowledge and skill in meeting participation or even facilitation; however, the expectation would be such that someone new did not need these skills until after the 90-day onboarding period. Additionally, information regarding accrediting and regulatory bodies, such as The Joint Commission and the Centers for Medicare and Medicaid Services, and even including Magnet Recognition from the American Nurses Credentialing Center, should be discussed, but again probably not until after the 90-day onboarding period.

- The final question might be one that many of you would want to pose first—what do we already have in place to support our new nurses? The advantage of asking this question last is that you are not boxed into the ways you have done things previously. By asking this first, you run head first into the wall of the existing orientation program and onboarding process. Answering this last allows you to answer the question from a different perspective, because the other questions have helped shape and change your expectations of your onboarding process.

These questions should be asked and answered by the principals—the key stakeholders in the process. We will have more on them later in this chapter.

Analysis/Design Principle 2: Be Clear about Job, Team, and Organizational Responsibilities

This should be easy to do, but is not as straightforward as you might think. You started with a job description that guided the hiring process. Most job descriptions include the ubiquitous "other duties as assigned." That leaves many questions unanswered for a new employee. Many larger facilities will have opportunities for nurses to serve beyond their daily job duties. Other duties may include serving on committees, collecting data for research projects, or serving as the chair for a fundraising campaign. Your new hires need to understand team and organizational responsibilities as well.

In addition to team and/or organizational goals (such as quality indicators or safety metrics), additional activities could include involvement in shared governance, improvement projects, and task forces, among others. If involvement in these groups is an expected behavior, that should be communicated clearly to the new employee along with *how* and *when* involvement begins.

Analysis/Design Principle 3: Leverage Appropriate Models

We have introduced you to the ADDIE model, and you will want to leverage other models to enhance your program. We have ones that we have found to be useful and we will spend more time on the models in Chapter 2, but we wanted to highlight that selecting the right models to use as you design and develop a program will be critical to its success. The ones we suggest are:

- Kolb's Experiential Learning Model
- Myers-Briggs Type Indicator (MBTI)
- VARK
- AACN Synergy Model for Patient Care™

Develop/Implement Principle 1: Engage the Employees Each and Every Day

Employee engagement is a buzz-phrase that is probably a bit overused; however, given the statistics we shared with you earlier in this chapter, we believe that engagement is important each and every day. In fact, by working with your Human Resources and/or Talent Acquisition team, you can engage your new employees before they even start working. The time between acceptance of a new job and starting the new job can be a challenging time for your new employees. Reach out to them, and start talking about the onboarding process. Let them know how excited you are to have them on the team. Engage, engage, engage. You can do this by talking on the phone, inviting them to coffee, sending an email with their agenda for the first few days of work, etc.

So, what exactly does engagement have to do with onboarding and orientation? Well, have you ever participated in an orientation program and felt like you were sitting in front of talking heads who were just there to regurgitate information for your "benefit"? If you can make orientation engaging, you will be less likely to lose people the first day. Try to make even the basic stuff interactive, and your new staff will love you and the job! For example, instead of simply lecturing through various policies and procedures, you could try using a case study approach where orientees break up into groups and are asked a series of guided questions that will require them to work through the policy and procedure manual. Or you can assign small groups certain key policies and procedures and have them "teach back" to the rest of the group. These are both more interactive methods to help new employees learn what can be a bit boring.

For the onboarding process, engagement should not really be an issue, but unfortunately, sometimes it is. In the book *How Full Is Your Bucket? Positive Strategies for Work and Life,* Tom Rath and Donald O. Clifton (2004) highlight the fact that disengagement costs U.S. businesses over $250 billion in lost productivity, illness, injuries, etc. And while it is not always about the money, most healthcare facilities want to have practices that will prevent them from losing money.

Did you know:

- The number one reason people leave their job is because they do not feel appreciated?

- Studies suggest that bad bosses can increase the risk of stroke by one-third?

- 90% of people say that they are more productive when they are around people with positive attitudes? (Rath & Clifton, 2004)

Engaging people is not difficult. To help with this problem, you can try applying the Golden Rule, "Do unto others as you would have them do unto you," or the more profound Platinum Rule, "Do unto others as they would have you do unto them." In other words, treat people the way they want to be treated. This means that you find preceptors who are really interested in teaching clinical skills. You identify nurse educators who have a passion for learning, teaching, and helping others grow. These people will help keep your new nurses engaged. And, most importantly, you take the time to get to know each person as an individual.

We know that some of this seems very basic. However, employee surveys would suggest that as leaders and educators, we sometimes fall down in the area of engagement. So, here are some simple things you can do to make sure that you are engaging your new nurses each and every day:

- Treat them with the respect they deserve, and they will reciprocate.

- Share the load—this person is not a nursing assistant. Do not ask them to do anything that you would not do.

- Answer questions in a respectful manner. Questions help people learn, and one of your most important roles is to help them learn.

- Make sure that you explain the "why" of a situation if it is not self-evident. Humans are meaning-making beings, and understanding the "why" of any situation helps people put it in the right context.

- If you are someone who keeps a busy schedule, go ahead and begin blocking off time in your calendar where you plan to simply check in with the new employee, whether that's in person or through an email or phone call.

Develop/Implement Principle 2: Provide (and Accept) Feedback Early and Often

Feedback is critical to success. It is critical to the success of your new nurses, and it is critical to the success of your onboarding program. That means that feedback is a two-way street. In order to facilitate that feedback, we want to introduce you to the EARS model. This model was codeveloped by the coauthor of this book Robin L. Jarvis and her colleague Debra R. France as a way for managers to provide employees with clear performance feedback. It has since been used as an interview methodology as well. The model (Table 1.1) can be used to give positive and constructive feedback.

TABLE 1.1 *The EARS Model*

MODEL	EXPLANATION	EXAMPLES
Example	A specific time or setting when the performance occurred (context)	*Positive or Constructive*—"When you were administering medication to Patient X…"
Action	The specific behavior or action the person took	*Positive*—"you followed our medication protocol exactly." *Constructive*—"you did not double-check the medicine against the electronic medical record, per our protocol."
Results	The implications of the behavior or action	*Positive*—"This ensured that the patient got the correct medication in the correct dosage." *Constructive*—"Although you did give the right medication in the right dosage, you could have given the wrong medication."
Suggestions	An opportunity for you and the employee to discuss what worked well or what the employee could do differently next time	*Positive*—"You seem to have the protocol down, but I wanted to see if you have any questions about it." *Constructive*—"What can you do next time to ensure that you follow the protocol? How can I help?"

Providing this level of feedback helps the new employee understand what he/she is doing well and what specifically he/she can improve. We recommend sharing this model with your new employees and asking them to provide feedback to you in a similar manner. Their feedback can help you improve your orientation program and your onboarding process.

Evaluation Principle 1: Base the Evaluation on the Program Objectives

How will you know if your onboarding program is successful? You will have to evaluate it. On what do you base the evaluation? You developed program objectives based on the analysis you do, so using those objectives is the best way to evaluate the success of your program. You will need to determine how to get the evaluation information. You might use a combination of surveys, anecdotal information, and feedback from participants, preceptors, and hiring managers. There are several models for evaluation. We go into greater detail about program evaluation in Chapter 6.

Evaluation Principle 2: Evaluate the Participants and the Program Regularly

Because the purpose of the onboarding program is to prepare your nurses to work independently in their assigned unit, you will need ways to evaluate the participants as well. In Chapter 4, we look in great detail at ways to evaluate individual competency; however, for now, we want to talk about what it means to evaluate the program and the participants regularly.

In the Analyze phase, we asked the question about what success looks like for a nurse at 30, 60, and 90 days. The answer to that question provides a great basis for evaluating individuals throughout the onboarding process. The preceptor and hiring manager should be providing the participant with regular feedback about his/her progress and competency level. Someone said that change is the only constant, and you should expect that with your onboarding program. At regular intervals perhaps once or twice per year you should evaluate the overall program. This will include what we discussed in Evaluation Principle 1, and we provide more suggestions for this in Chapter 6.

Principals

Principals are the people who are stakeholders in the orientation program and the onboarding process. They may include:

- Hiring manager
- Nurse educator
- Preceptor

- Unit nursing director
- Hospital/organizational nursing director
- Other healthcare providers
- Patient(s) and family
- New employee

Each principal will bring unique insights, experiences, and ideas to the party. Getting input from all of them will help ensure that you understand their expectations for the onboarding process. Obviously, this list was made from the perspective of a good-sized hospital. You will need to adjust your list of principals based on the requirements and structure of your organization. There will be different ways of engaging the stakeholders to get their input as well.

The hiring manager, the nurse educator, and the preceptor probably have the biggest stakes in ensuring the success of the new employee. The good news is that you probably have gathered their input if you applied Analysis/Design Principle 1 (answering the right questions) successfully. The questions from Principle 1 cannot be answered in a vacuum, so if you sought input, it was likely from these three people.

Specific information you can glean from the hiring manager should hit all of the principles highlighted earlier. The hiring manager should be able to articulate job expectations and responsibilities, how success is measured, and how frequently feedback will be provided. You may also bring in peers and other healthcare providers (such as physicians or ancillary staff) at this point to discuss what level of competence is required to independently and safely care for patients.

The nurse educator and preceptor are two sides of the same coin. Ideally, the preceptor is providing coaching and feedback on clinical skills in real time, and the nurse educator is facilitating sessions to help the new nurse be a better leader by focusing on some of the socio-emotional skills required to be successful. Although the educator may be found teaching clinical skills, this will likely be done in a simulated or classroom session.

Unit and organizational directors can provide "high-level" insight into how the mission and vision of the organization influences the expectations of an orientation program. Because organizations are constantly changing, these principals need to assess the current state of—and determine the future direction for—an orientation program as it relates to the organization's goals.

Conclusion

Remember, you have invested a lot of time and money to bring new nurses into your organization. Developing a great onboarding and orientation program will help ensure that your investment pays off. By applying the concepts presented in this chapter, you are well on your way to having an onboarding approach that is engaging and rewarding and one that will keep your new nurses excited about their roles in your organization.

Questions for Reflection/Discussion

1. Who are your principals for this onboarding program?
2. What are your next steps in working on the onboarding program?
3. If time and resources were not an issue, what would your ideal nursing orientation and onboarding program look like?

KEY TAKEAWAYS

- *Onboard, don't overboard your new nurses!*
- *Apply the ADDIE model principles to make your process and program a success.*
- *Engage the principals early and often.*

References

Branson, R. K., Rayner, G. T., Cox, J. L., Furman, J. P., King, F. J., & Hannum, W. H. (1975). *Interservice procedures for instructional systems development.* (5 vols.) (TRADOC Pam 350-30 NAVEDTRA 106A). Ft. Monroe, VA: U.S. Army Training and Doctrine Command, August 1975. (NTIS No. ADA 019 486 through ADA 019 490).

France, D., & Jarvis, L. (1996, October). Quick starts for new employees. *Training & Development, 50*(10), 47-50.

Freeman, D. (2013). *Onboarding and socialization for better retention.* Emeryville, CA: Cytiva, Inc.

Laurano, M. (2013). *Onboarding 2013: A new look at new hires.* Aberdeen Group. Retrieved from http://pages.silkroad.com/rs/silkroad/images/Onboarding-2013-A-NewLook-at-New-Hires-Aberdeen.pdf?mkt_tok=3RkMMJWWfF9wsRovsq%2FMZKXonj HpfsX87%2B4oXaK0lMI%2F0ER3fOvrPUfGjI4ARMNqMa%2B TFAwTG5toziV8R7TNL810w9AQWhPm

Rath, T., & Clifton, D. O. (2004). *How full is your bucket? Positive strategies for work and life.* New York, NY: Gallup Press.

Schein, E. (2009). *The corporate culture survival guide.* San Francisco, CA: Jossey-Bass.

CHAPTER 2

Analyzing and Designing an Orientation Program

Introduction

Now that you have some basic understanding of the approach and the key principles and principals, it's time to take a deeper look at the Analysis and Design phases of the project that you started looking at in Chapter 1. To really analyze what you've got in a program and what you want and to position yourself to design a successful program you need to:

- Collect data from the principals

- Assess any existing programs

- Understand your learners

- Consider how culture and connection will fit into your program structure

Only when you have taken these steps are you ready to make recommendations and move to design.

Gathering Data From the Principals

You'll remember from Chapter 1 that principals are the key people who need to be involved in the development, implementation, and sustainability of the program. There are various ways to collect the information you need from them. However, you will want to adjust your data-gathering method based on the principal involved. Table 2.1 highlights some data-gathering techniques and with whom you might wish to use them.

TABLE 2.1 *Data-Gathering Methods*

METHOD	EXPLANATION	PRINCIPALS
One-on-One Interviews	This method provides the greatest amount of anecdotal information; however, it can be very time consuming.	Unit/organizational directors
Focus Groups	This method can be a great way to gather a lot of information. We recommend that if you use focus groups, you separate them by stakeholder group. Your groups should have at least five people and no more than nine or ten.	Hiring managers, preceptors, nurse educators, other healthcare providers, new employees
Survey	Surveys can be used effectively if you have a large number of people and little time. They can be used to collect information from a more disparate group of individuals.	Patients and families, new employees

Interview Questions

When interviewing unit or organizational directors, you'll want to be sure to cover certain key areas by asking the following:

- What does success look like for a nurse on your unit?

- What are the most important behaviors you want to see from a nurse on your unit?

- What are the most important things (projects, success factors, etc.) that a new nurse on your unit needs to know?

- Whom do they need to know?

You'll want to tailor other questions to your specific situation, but these listed questions represent ground you'll definitely want to cover.

So, You Want to Run a Focus Group...

If you are planning on using a focus group, Table 2.2 provides a suggested agenda as well as some facilitation ideas that you can apply. We recommend that your focus group have no more than eight to ten participants, and you should allow 90 minutes for the meeting. This agenda would work well with hiring managers, nurse educators, and preceptors.

TABLE 2.2 *Focus Group Agenda*

TOPIC	WHO	HOW	TIME/TOTAL
Welcome	Facilitator	Discuss purpose Review agenda Review ground rules Introductions (if needed)	15 minutes/ 15 minutes
What does success look like?	All	Groups of 3 –Discuss –Capture ideas on flipcharts Large group –Group reports –Discuss –Agree	30 minutes/ 45 minutes
Whom do they need to know?	All	Thought gallery –1 flipchart each for 30, 60, and 90 days –Each participant gets sticky notes –One idea per sticky note –Placed on appropriate flipchart –Discuss –Agree	30 minutes/ 75 minutes
What else do they need to know?	All	Discuss (capture on flipchart)	10 minutes/ 85 minutes
Next steps	Facilitator	Share with group Thank them for their participation	5 minutes/ 90 minutes

Conducting Surveys

You'll use surveys most often to gather information from patients and families and from new employees. Before we talk about survey questions, we want to talk about survey tools you can use, and what you need to know about writing surveys in general.

Most people are connected to the Internet, so we would recommend using an electronic survey tool. Many of these are inexpensive, or possibly even free, depending upon how often you want to survey, how many people you want to survey, and how much analytical support you will need. Some possible tools include:

- SurveyMonkey—https://www.surveymonkey.com/

- SoGoSurvey—http://www.sogosurvey.com/

- FluidSurveys—http://fluidsurveys.com/

Once you have selected a tool to use and are ready to start writing the survey, here are a few suggestions that can make your survey easy to read, easy to complete, and useful for you.

- Have you heard of KISS—Keep It Simple, Silly? Surveys are no exception to this adage. Ideally, keep it to no more than 2 to 3 electronic pages, with no more than 10 to 12 questions per page. If it is longer than that (and 3 pages with 12 questions is getting pretty long), people will be less likely to complete it.

- Primarily count on scale-based questions, with a few open-ended questions at the end. If possible, use the same scale throughout the survey. Here are a couple of scales that seem to work:

  - 0 Not applicable 1 Disagree completely 2 Disagree
    3 Neutral 4 Agree 5 Agree completely

  - 0 Not applicable 1 Dislike completely 2 Dislike 3 Neither
    Like nor Dislike 4 Like 5 Like completely

- Offer an out for the participant. Note that the scales above include a 0 for Not applicable. Give people the opportunity to not answer the question if it doesn't fit their experiences.

- When writing a scale-based question, make it a statement. For example, "The care I received from the nursing staff was consistent."

- Avoid questions that ask more than one thing at time. You would not want to use, "The care I received from the nursing staff was consistent and they treated me with dignity and respect." These are two separate items.

- Use open-ended questions sparingly. Great questions to use include, "What did you like best about X?" or "What did you like least about X?" and "What would you do to make X better?" These allow the participant to provide meaningful feedback.

Finally, here are some questions you might want to ask a couple of groups impacted by the onboarding program recent orientees and the patients and families they treated.

Sample questions for current and recent orientees:

- I received the training I needed to be successful on my unit.

- I met the people I needed to know to be successful in my job.

- I can articulate the expectations of this job.

- I know what the organization's mission is.

- I know what the organization's vision is.

- I can complete key procedures needed for patients on this unit.

- What did I need to know that I did not learn?

- What else would I have liked to know?

- I recommend that the following changes be considered…

Sample questions for patients and families:

- I was treated with dignity and respect.

- I received competent care from the nursing staff.

- I received consistent care from the nursing staff.

- I would recommend this facility to others.

Assessing Strengths and Weaknesses of Existing Program

If you have a program already, this section is for you. If not, you may wish to skip to the next section of the chapter.

Assessing the strengths and weaknesses of an existing program starts with Analysis, just like the ADDIE model shows us. Chapter 1 refers to key questions that must be asked as you design a program. You can ask those same questions and then compare your existing program to the answers. As a reminder, here are those questions:

- Who are the learners and what are their commonalities and differences?

- What behaviors and skills do you want to see them execute successfully?

- What constraints exist that may prevent them from performing successfully?

- What methods will you employ to help them learn and practice?

- What adult learning theories might you need to apply throughout the program?

- What existing content and/or materials do you have?

- What is your timeline for completion?

The second thing you should do is look at the learning objectives of the program. Dr. John Sullivan, one of HR's "Top 10 Leading Thinkers," has developed 15 common errors to avoid in onboarding programs (Sullivan, 2008). One way to assess the strengths and weaknesses of your program is to use his common errors as filters. We have reduced the number of the errors he suggests by combining like errors. So, using Table 2.3 adapted from Dr. Sullivan's work, you can determine the strengths and potential weaknesses of your existing program.

TABLE 2.3 *Common Errors to Avoid in Onboarding Programs*

ERROR	BRIEF DESCRIPTION	POTENTIAL ACTIONS TO TAKE
Overloading new employees on day one	Providing too much information in a non-interactive manner	Use electronic tools for HR issues such as benefits enrollment, etc. Intersperse presentations with engaging videos of executives and other employees
Being rigid about the time frame	Viewing onboarding as the first day or two at work. Onboarding should last 6 to 12 months	Use a competency-based approach to ensure that each new nurse gets the right amount of tutelage and supervision

ERROR	BRIEF DESCRIPTION	POTENTIAL ACTIONS TO TAKE
Forgetting to take an integrated approach	Focusing only on organizational level, or unit level, rather than including team, individual, and/or department level	HR should provide the organizational level Hiring manager, nurse educator, and/or preceptor provides the unit, team, and individual level onboarding
One-way communication	Asking for little or no input from the new nurse	Ensure that new nurse has opportunity to ask questions and provide feedback on the process
No metrics or accountability	Providing no measures of success at any level of the program	Develop metrics that address things such as retention, hiring manager participation in onboarding, individual time to productivity, etc.
Ignoring diverse needs	Failing to acknowledge that your new nurses have different levels of experience, knowledge, and skills	Use a competency-based approach to ensure that each new nurse gets the right amount of tutelage and supervision
Manager's expectations are unclear and presence is lacking	Ensuring that the manager is present, communicates expectations, and stays in touch with the nurse educator, preceptor, and new nurse	Develop a checklist for hiring managers that provides check-in times/opportunities Ensure that the nurse educator and preceptor communicate regularly with the hiring manager
Lack of business case	Senior leaders (unit directors and above) do not understand the criticality of onboarding	Build a business case Keep it current with metrics from your program Get it in front of new leaders as soon as possible
Failure to reinforce the organizational brand	New employees do not recognize the value that your organization provides in the community and they can't articulate it to others	Ensure that the HR session includes corporate values, corporate responsibility platform, etc. Have new hires practice a short (15- to 30-second) response to, "Why did you choose to work for X?"
Delays in offering onboarding	Asking new employees to wait until a certain number of new employees are available	Hold start dates until you have the right number of participants This may be more relevant for new college graduate nurses than experienced nurses

Adapted from Sullivan, 2008

So, now that you've gathered all this data from your principals and you've assessed what is and isn't working in your current program (if you have one), what do you do next? You take this information and analyze it so you can:

1. Come to some understanding about your learners

2. Consider what you need from your program from a 30,000-foot perspective

3. Develop some recommendations

The next sections dig into these three important steps.

Understanding Your Learners

Before you dive into all the ins and outs of orientation and onboarding programs, you need to spend some time talking about the people who will be going through your program—your new nurses. And in the context of orientation and onboarding, you can more accurately look at them as your *learners*. We want to make sure that you keep your learners in mind during the entire process. To do that, you have to understand how they process information and translate that into learning. There are many learning style models and theories out there, but we want to focus on just a handful that are easy to understand and translate into actions you can take as you build and implement your program.

- Kolb's Experiential Learning Model

- Myers-Briggs Type Indicator (MBTI)

- VARK Information Processing Model

In addition to these three learning models, to consider the connection of nurse practice to patient and family outcomes as you design your program, we encourage the use of the AACN Synergy Model for Patient Care™.

Kolb's Experiential Learning Model

The first learning style model we will discuss is David A. Kolb's (1984) model for experiential learning (McLeod, 2013). This model will provide a great foundation for you, as many of your new employees will (a) be accustomed to experiential learning and (b) prefer it as a way to develop efficacy. Essentially, the model suggests four simple steps—that a person should:

1. Experience something

2. Be able to think about what he/she has experienced

3. Draw from that experience some knowledge or learning

4. Have an opportunity to apply the learning in a new and different way.

Figure 2.1 illustrates Kolb's model, and the accompanying Table 2.4 explains the steps along with an example of administering an intravenous medication for the first time.

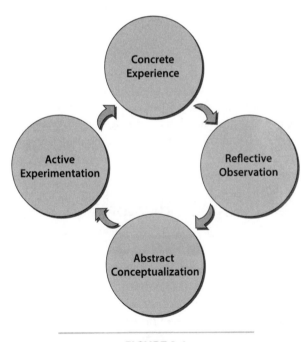

FIGURE 2.1

Kolb's Experiential Learning Model.

TABLE 2.4 *Kolb's Experiential Learning Model*

STEP	BRIEF DESCRIPTION	EXAMPLE
Concrete Experience	Doing or having an experience	The learner observes the preceptor administering an intravenous (IV) analgesic to a hospitalized patient experiencing pain.
Reflective Observation	Reflecting on and reviewing the experience	After observing the preceptor, the learner reflects on (thinks about) the event and the details involved.
Abstract Concept-ualization	Drawing conclusions or learning from the experience	The learner begins to analyze and understand why the medication was given, why the IV route was chosen, how quickly the patient responded, how the preceptor organized the supplies, etc.
Active Experi-mentation	Trying out what has been learned	The next day, the learner attempts administration of an IV analgesic to a patient experiencing pain.

Keeping Kolb's model for experiential learning in front of you as you plan onboarding for your learners will mean paying attention to making the process experiential, while giving learners the opportunity to reflect and understand how they can take the learning and apply it in different settings.

Myers-Briggs Type Indicator (MBTI)

The second learning theory or model we will discuss is the Myers-Briggs Type Indicator (MBTI). Robin has been a qualified administrator and interpreter of the MBTI for over 15 years. This instrument was developed by the mother and daughter team of Katherine Cook Briggs and Isabel Briggs Myers and is based on the work of Carl Jung. There are four dichotomies in the MBTI, which allow for a possible combination of 16 types. Rather than chronicle the learning style specifics for all 16 types, we want to provide an overview of the dichotomies and address how these affect learning in Table 2.5. We are providing some definitions, as some of the words are not used in MBTI-speak as they are in regular conversation (The Myers-Briggs Foundation, 2013).

TABLE 2.5 *Myers-Briggs Type Indicator*

MAJOR AREAS	DICHOTOMIES	BRIEF DEFINITIONS	LEARNING EXAMPLES
Energy	Extrovert (E)	Draws energy from being with others. Talks to think.	Usually likes role playing and large group activities.
	Introvert (I)	Draws energy from being alone or in small groups. Thinks, then speaks.	Usually needs time to think before speaking and prefers small group activities.
Information Gathering	Sensing (S)	Gathers information through five senses. Likes details.	Likes the big picture and takes information to form patterns.
	Intuition (N)	Likes processes and wants information in the correct order.	Needs the big picture in order for the details to fit.
Decision Making	Thinking (T)	Makes decisions based on data and logic.	Prefers activities that include the data.
	Feeling (F)	Makes decisions based on values and impact on others.	Prefers activities that are people- or values-oriented.
Lifestyle	Judging (J)	Likes to make decisions and move to next item.	Prefers to leave things open-ended in case more information is available.
	Perceiving (P)	Likes activities that require decisive action.	Likes activities in which gathering data is more important than the decision.

The MBTI concepts are not only important when considering *your* presentation of material in a setting such as a classroom but also when selecting preceptors for your orientees. For example, if preceptors and orientees have fundamentally different approaches to decision-making (such as one being predominantly thinking while the other being predominantly feeling), the preceptor may perceive that the orientee is unable to make good decisions in the clinical setting. In reality, both approaches are valid (and some may be more appropriate in some situations than others, such as during end-of-life care), but there are fundamental differences between the teacher and learner.

VARK Information Processing Model

Another model that plays well into the design and implementation of any program is VARK. Developed by Neil Fleming, VARK stands for Visual, Aural, Read/Write, and Kinesthetic (Penn State Learning Design Community Hub, 2010). It is a model that addresses how people process information most effectively and indicates how a person prefers to receive information. In Table 2.6, we provide insights into how to leverage VARK.

TABLE 2.6 *VARK Information Processing Model*

PREFERENCE	BRIEF DEFINITION	LEARNING EXAMPLES
Visual	Receives information by seeing it. Processes information quickly. Likes graphics.	Flipcharts and other visual aids help. Do not move visual aids to new locations (for visual learners, this is like shaking an Etch-a-Sketch).
Auditory	Receives information by hearing it…and being able to talk about it.	Tolerates "lectures" better than most; however, must be able to discuss what he/she has learned in order to cement the learning.
Reading-Writing	Processes information by reading it and writing about it.	May be willing to read aloud in class. Will want time to reflect and write in a learning journal.
Kinesthetic	Learns by doing and/or being emotionally attached to what is presented.	Let them "just do it!" When possible, help them feel the emotional connection of what they are doing.

A note about VARK—ideally, a well-developed program incorporates all four of these styles. Most people have a preference, but can process information via the other preferences as well. Only a few of your learners will require information be presented in their preferred way in order to comprehend the content. So, if you provide learning opportunities that incorporate all four preferences, your program should be successful and your learners should learn a great deal. For example, if you were teaching a class on the application of physical restraints for patients with psychiatric illnesses, you may want to present information in more ways than simply lecturing with a PowerPoint presentation (auditory and visual styles). You may consider incorporating time to practice the application of restraints (kinesthetic), as well as delivering a written case study requiring short-answer responses regarding the topic of ethical and legal considerations (reading-writing).

Of course, there are many other theories and models for how people learn; however, we believe that these three can have a significant positive impact in the development and implementation of the program and, most importantly, the self-efficacy of your learners.

AACN Synergy Model for Patient Care

Although it would be a great idea to include representation from patients and their families when making decisions about orientation design, it may be difficult to facilitate their presence at these meetings. Therefore, we propose using the American Association of Critical-Care Nurses (AACN) Synergy Model for Patient Care in consideration of the needs of patients and families, as it was designed to assist in demonstrating the connection between a nurse's practice and the patient's outcomes (AACN.org, 2013).

The AACN Synergy Model looks at matching patient/family needs and the characteristics and competencies of nurses. According to AACN.org (2013), "Synergy results when the needs and characteristics of a patient, clinical unit or system are matched with a nurse's competencies." So, how does this impact the design of an onboarding program?

Based on the type of patients and the care your unit is providing, you will need a certain level of competency. This should inform the length of onboarding and the type of additional training needed, as well as help you to identify critical success factors for your nurses. Check out Table 2.7 for more information on the various components of the Synergy Model.

TABLE 2.7 *Definitions of the AACN Synergy Model Characteristics of Patients, Clinical Units, and Systems*

CHARACTERISTIC	DESCRIPTION
Resiliency	The capacity to return to a restorative level of functioning using compensatory/coping mechanisms; the ability to bounce back quickly after an insult
Vulnerability	Susceptibility to actual or potential stressors that may adversely affect patient outcomes
Stability	The ability to maintain a steady-state equilibrium
Complexity	The intricate entanglement of two or more systems (e.g., body, family, therapies)
Resource availability	Extent of resources (e.g., technical, fiscal, personal, psychological, and social) the patient/family/ community brings to the situation
Participation in care	Extent to which patient/family engages in aspects of care
Participation in decision-making	Extent to which patient/family engages in decision-making
Predictability	A characteristic that allows one to expect a certain course of events or course of illness

Source: AACN.org, 2013. Information in tables is retrieved from http://www.aacn. org/wd/certifications/content/synmodel.pcms. Used with permission.

Table 2.8 provides definitions of the nurse competencies from the Synergy Model. These competencies were developed to illustrate how nurses can effectively meet the needs of patients. Therefore, these components could be the organizing framework by which hiring managers and unit directors set expectations of their onboarding program.

TABLE 2.8 *Definitions of the AACN Synergy Model Nurse Competencies*

CHARACTERISTIC	DESCRIPTION
Clinical Judgment	Clinical reasoning, which includes clinical decision-making, critical thinking, and a global grasp of the situation, coupled with nursing skills acquired through a process of integrating formal and informal experiential knowledge and evidence-based guidelines
Advocacy and Moral Agency	Working on another's behalf and representing the concerns of the patient/family and nursing staff; serving as a moral agent in identifying and helping to resolve ethical and clinical concerns within and outside the clinical setting
Caring Practices	Nursing activities that create a compassionate, supportive, and therapeutic environment for patients and staff, with the aim of promoting comfort and healing and preventing unnecessary suffering. Includes, but is not limited to, vigilance, engagement, and responsiveness of caregivers, including family and healthcare personnel
Collaboration	Working with others (for example, patients, families, healthcare providers) in a way that promotes/encourages each person's contributions toward achieving optimal/realistic patient/family goals; involves intra- and interdisciplinary work with colleagues and community
Systems Thinking	Body of knowledge and tools that allow the nurse to manage whatever environmental and system resources exist for the patient/family and staff, within or across healthcare and non-healthcare systems
Response to Diversity	The sensitivity to recognize, appreciate, and incorporate differences into the provision of care; differences may include, but are not limited to, cultural differences, spiritual beliefs, gender, race, ethnicity, lifestyle, socioeconomic status, age, and values
Facilitation of Learning	The ability to facilitate learning for patients/families, nursing staff, other members of the healthcare team and community; includes both formal and informal facilitation of learning
Clinical Inquiry (Innovator/Evaluator)	The ongoing process of questioning and evaluating practice and providing informed practice; creating practice changes through research utilization and experiential learning

Source: AACN.org, 2013. Information in tables is retrieved from http://www.aacn.org/wd/certifications/content/synmodel.pcms. Used with permission.

In addition, to bring the definitions of these competencies to life, the AACN also provides a few examples of what behaviors a nurse may exhibit depending on what degree of competency (using some of Patricia Benner's levels) the nurse has achieved. Benner's (1982, 2004) Novice to Expert theory outlines a continuum of increasing nurse competency that starts with Novice and Advanced Beginner. The Synergy Model rates nurses on a scaled continuum of 1-5, where a 1 corresponds to Benner's Competent stage that follows Advanced Beginner (see Chapter 4 for more information on Benner's theory). Nurses completing orientation are likely somewhere between the Advanced Beginner and Competent stages, so for purposes of this text, we have chosen to list only the first level as it represents the minimum level of competency that most would agree is needed to independently provide care. Table 2.9 provides these Level 1 characteristics.

TABLE 2.9 *Level 1 Characteristics of the AACN Synergy Model Nurse Competencies*

CHARACTERISTIC	DESCRIPTION
Clinical Judgment	Collects basic-level data; follows algorithms, decision trees, and protocols with all populations and is uncomfortable deviating from them; matches formal knowledge with clinical events to make decisions; questions the limits of one's ability to make clinical decisions and delegates the decision-making to other clinicians; includes extraneous detail
Advocacy and Moral Agency	Works on behalf of patient; self-assesses personal values; aware of ethical conflicts/issues that may surface in clinical setting; makes ethical/moral decisions based on rules; represents patient when patient cannot represent self; aware of patients' rights
Caring Practices	Focuses on the usual and customary needs of the patient; no anticipation of future needs; bases care on standards and protocols; maintains a safe physical environment; acknowledges death as a potential outcome
Collaboration	Willing to be taught, coached and/or mentored; participates in team meetings and discussions regarding patient care and/or practice issues; open to various team members' contributions
Systems Thinking	Uses a limited array of strategies; limited outlook—sees the pieces or components; does not recognize negotiation as an alternative; sees patient and family within the isolated environment of the unit; sees self as key resource
Response to Diversity	Assesses cultural diversity; provides care based on own belief system; learns the culture of the healthcare environment

CHARACTERISTIC	DESCRIPTION
Facilitation of Learning	Follows planned educational programs; sees patient/family education as a separate task from delivery of care; provides data without seeking to assess patient's readiness or understanding; has limited knowledge of the totality of the educational needs; focuses on a nurse's perspective; sees the patient as a passive recipient
Clinical Inquiry (Innovator/ Evaluator)	Follows standards and guidelines; implements clinical changes and research-based practices developed by others; recognizes the need for further learning to improve patient care; recognizes obvious changing patient situation (e.g., deterioration, crisis); needs and seeks help to identify patient problem

Source: AACN.org, 2013. Information in tables is retrieved from http://www.aacn.org/wd/ certifications/content/synmodel.pcms. Used with permission.

It can be tempting to expect a new hire to perform at the same degree of competency as an experienced nurse in the organization, and the AACN Synergy Model can assist in designing a program that ensures basic competency without setting unrealistic expectations. While the discussion on assessing an individual's competency will come in Chapter 4, part of designing a successful orientation program is setting targets that are achievable, and the AACN Synergy Model may help you do just that.

Program Structure and the Four C's of Onboarding

Now that we have discussed the learner (the new employee) as the ultimate focus of our orientation and onboarding program, let's jump to a 30,000-foot perspective of orientation and onboarding. Talya M. Bauer, PhD (2012), has developed a model (Figure 2.2) for successful onboarding known as the Four C's. These are the building blocks for self-efficacy for your new employees.

Keeping Bauer's model in mind as you consider design, development, and implementation elements will be critical in ensuring a strong orientation and onboarding program for your new nurses. Many programs do not include more than compliance and clarification; however, programs that include the culture and connection aspects will end up with more knowledgeable and engaged nursing staff. Including culture and connection should also improve retention of your new employees, because those levels provide more support on a personal and organizational level. The more that your new employees understand about the organization and what it stands for, the more likely they will be to work to support those values. Connection cannot be overrated either. In the book *Vital Friends* (2006), Tom Rath's research suggested that "[w]hile most companies spend their time thinking about how to increase an employee's loyalty to their organization, our research suggest they might want to find a different approach: *fostering the kind of loyalty that is built between one employee and another.* This is what keeps people in their jobs" (p. 58).

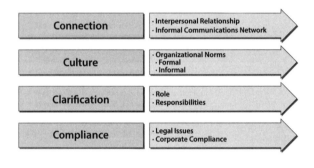

FIGURE 2.2

The Four C's of Onboarding.
(Information in figure taken from Bauer, 2012. Used with permission.)

Making Recommendations

Now that you've reviewed the existing program, looked at your learners and their needs, and interviewed the key principals, you are ready to pull the information together and start making recommendations. If appropriate, you should make recommendations at the organizational and unit levels. Your recommendations should be presented to the key principals, with the exception of the new nurses, patients, and families.

You will develop a PowerPoint deck with your recommendations, if that makes sense in your organizational culture. If not, you might develop a short paper that highlights your key findings and the recommendations you are making. A suggested outline for the PowerPoint or the paper would be:

- **Methodology**—This should include the data-gathering process, as well as who participated

- **Key Findings**—Based on the data gathered, what did you discover? This is an opportunity to introduce them to Bauer's model (Figure 2.2) and tie your findings to the four elements of the model.

- **Proposed Learning Objectives**—This will allow the key principals to see what you plan to accomplish with the program and will make your recommendations easier to understand.

- **Recommendations**—Given the findings, how do you propose that the organization and/or unit should proceed? Again, you have an opportunity to tie your recommendations to Bauer's model. Don't forget to tie them to the learning objectives, too!

- **Call to Action/Next Steps**—What do you need from the key principals to proceed? Who will be involved, how much do you think it will cost, and how long will it take? These are the questions that your key principals will want to know.

Figures 2.3 and 2.4 show a couple of sample slides that might be in a recommendation slide deck.

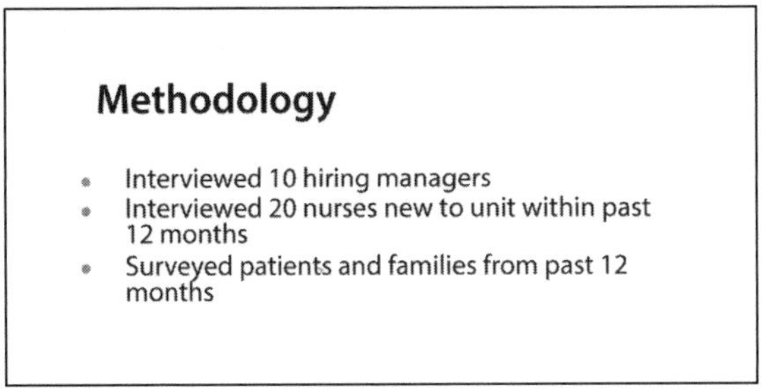

FIGURE 2.3

Recommendation slide example 1.

Recommendations

- Develop 3–6 month onboarding process
- Include organizational level orientation
- Provide preceptor support
- Hire in cohorts to establish support network early
- Implement in Q2 next year

FIGURE 2.4

Recommendation slide example 2.

Designing the Program

Now that your recommendations have been approved, it's time to start working on the actual design of the onboarding program. You will want to review the big picture of your onboarding program and then start diving into each module, one at a time.

Over the years, we have used different worksheets to help us think through the design process. We have taken the best of the worksheets and put them together for you. As you begin the design, you will want to create design worksheets for each module. Also, you might create a metaworksheet that highlights the overall goals of your onboarding program. When you have finished with design, you will have multiple worksheets. Worksheet Template 2.1 is a suggested worksheet for your use.

We wanted to provide you with a couple of examples as well. Sample Worksheet 2.1 looks at an organizational-level module on effective communication skills, and Sample Worksheet 2.2 addresses a unit-level module.

Conclusion

If you take the time to analyze and design your program, the rest will come more easily. Take your learning objectives and turn them into design worksheets. This will make the development and implementation a little easier because you have the information you need for each module at your fingertips! You do not have to reinvent the wheel, discover fire, or develop a better lightbulb! You have access to the AACN Synergy Model and other information that can guide what your orientation and onboarding program should be. In Chapter 3, we will help you take those design worksheets and begin to turn them into PowerPoint slides, facilitator notes, and Participant Guides. Let's go!

WORKSHEET TEMPLATE 2.1 *Design Worksheet*

Target Population Description			
Learning Objectives			
Delivery System(s) (Instructor-led, Simulations, etc.)			
Existing Content and/or Models and Theories to Use			
Materials Needed			
Sequence of Instruction (and Duration)	Topic	Method	Duration
Evaluation Method (should tie back to learning objectives and program goals)	Program: How will we measure the effectiveness of the program? Individual: How will we assess the new nurse as he/she moves through orientation?		

SAMPLE WORKSHEET 2.1 *Organization-Level Module*

Target Population Description	New college graduate nurses		
Learning Objectives	By the end of this workshop, participants will be able to: Use an effective communications and delivery model to plan communications and select communication media; Present data and information effectively; Develop and deliver communications that positively influence others		
Delivery System(s) (Instructor-led, Simulations, etc.)	Instructor-led with multiple practice opportunities		
Existing Content and/or Models and Theories to Use	Joe Smith's presentation to AACN (May, 2013) *Crucial Conversations* by Patterson, Grenny, McMillan, Switzler, & Roppe *Leading with Questions* by Marquardt		
Materials Needed	PowerPoint deck with content loaded on laptop, Participant Guide, evaluation forms, name tents, flipcharts with easel, markers, LCD projector with screen		
Sequence of Instruction (and Duration)	Topic	Method	Duration
	Welcome	Discuss Introductory Activity	15 minutes
	Effective Communications	Mini-lecture Examples Your own case	30 minutes
	Influencing Effectively	Mini-lecture Examples Your own case	30 minutes
	Bringing It All Together	Prepare your case Practice with others Receive feedback	30 minutes
	Next Steps	Reflection Share	15 minutes
Evaluation Method (should tie back to learning objectives and program goals)	Program: How will we measure the effectiveness of the program? Participants are 95% satisfied (Level 1 evaluation) Their managers see improved communication and influence skills within 30 days (Level 3 evaluation) Individual: How will we assess the new nurse as he/she moves through orientation? Participant is able to communicate and influence in a classroom setting using his/her own communication skills. (Level 2 evaluation)		

SAMPLE WORKSHEET 2.2 *Unit-Level Module*

Target Population Description	Experienced nurses new to a critical care environment		
Learning Objectives	By the end of this workshop, participants will be able to: Identify "red flags" of impending shock; Describe common troubleshooting strategies for arterial pressure and central venous pressure (CVP) monitoring devices; Compare and contrast select inotropes and vasopressors		
Delivery System(s) (Instructor-led, Simulations, etc.)	Electronic module and Skills lab		
Existing Content and/or Models and Theories to Use	Unit-specific case studies *Essentials of Critical Care Orientation* (AACN)		
Materials Needed	IV tubing & fluids; Pressure transducers; Patient monitor; Manikins, low-fidelity; Whiteboard & markers		
Sequence of Instruction (and Duration)	Topic	Method	Duration
	"Red Flags" of Shock	Online Module	Prework
	Introduction	Presentation of Case Study	15 minutes
	Troubleshooting Arterial & CVP devices	Didactic Lecture Demonstration Hands-On Practice	30 minutes
	Inotropes & Vasopressors	Didactic Lecture Low-fidelity simulation	30 minutes
	Wrap-up	Group Discussion Paper Evaluation	15 minutes
Evaluation Method (should tie back to learning objectives and program goals)	Program: How will we measure the effectiveness of the program? Participants are 95% satisfied (Level 1 evaluation) Their preceptors see enhanced ability to manage patients with arterial & CVP transducers as well as patients experiencing shock (Level 3 evaluation) Individual: How will we assess the new nurse as he/she moves through orientation? Participant is able to demonstrate appropriate actions during the class's simulation & case study (Level 2 evaluation)		

Questions for Reflection/Discussion

1. Who needs to approve the recommendations and provide the budget for this program?

2. What is the best way to present your findings and recommendations?

3. Who will help you with the design of the program?

KEY TAKEAWAYS

- *The old adage "garbage in, garbage out" is something to keep in mind while doing your analysis. Make sure that you have the right people engaged and are asking the right questions.*

- *You must understand how your learners learn in order to teach effectively. By using the models highlighted in this chapter, you should reach almost all your learners!*

- *Use the design worksheet—one for each module. This will help you stay organized as you get ready to develop the materials.*

References

AACN.org. (2013). AACN synergy model for patient care. Retrieved from http://www.aacn.org/wd/certifications/content/synmodel.pcms

Bauer, T. M. (2012). *Onboarding new employees: Maximizing success* (SHRM Foundation Effective Practice Guidelines Series). Alexandria, VA: SHRM Foundation.

Benner, P. (1982). From novice to expert. *The American Journal of Nursing, 82*(3), 402-407.

Benner, P. (2004). Using the Dreyfus model of skill acquisition to describe and interpret skill acquisition and clinical judgment in nursing practice and education. *Bulletin of Science, Technology, & Society, 24*(3), 188-199.

McLeod, S. (2013). Kolb – learning styles. Retrieved from http://www.simplypsychology.org/learning-kolb.html

The Myers-Briggs Foundation. (2013). MBTI basics. Retrieved from http://www.myersbriggs.org/my-mbti-personality-type/mbti-basics/

Penn State Learning Design Community Hub. (2010). Learning Styles. Retrieved from http://ets.tlt.psu.edu/learningdesign/audience/learningstyles

Rath, T. (2006). *Vital friends: The people you can't afford to live without.* New York, NY: Gallup Press.

Sullivan, J. (2008, November 17). Onboarding program killers: 15 common errors to avoid. Retrieved from http://www.ere.net/2008/11/17/onboarding-program-killers-15-common-errors-to-avoid/

CHAPTER 3

Developing and Implementing an Orientation Program

Introduction

Some of you reading this book have the advantage of having an orientation and onboarding program already in place. Some of you do not, and that's why you picked up this book. Regardless of your situation, this chapter will help you develop and implement your orientation program. We will look at how to evaluate an existing program, organizational versus unit orientations, and then get into the anatomy of an orientation program for your new nurses.

Developing a Program

In Chapter 1, we introduced you to the ADDIE model. In Chapter 2, we walked you through how to analyze the onboarding situation as well as how to design by using design worksheets for each module of the program you want to create. Now you are going to use these worksheets to provide a road map for each particular learning module. Without this road map, you risk ending up at an undesired destination. Once the module has been created, you must develop any and all materials that you need to help your orientee learn. Using the examples we have provided here, let's talk about what you would do next.

The approach we have used in the past is as follows:

1. Review available content

2. Identify which content to use

3. Determine methods to present material and provide practice

4. Develop necessary supporting materials

The organizational level module in this example is about effective communication skills. Let's pretend we have identified some existing content from a presentation that Nurse Joe gave at XYZ conference in May of last year, as well as two books we believe have good insights and tools for effective communication. We have decided which content to use and have contacted Joe to make sure he is okay with us using some of his PowerPoint slides.

As we determine methods to present the material and provide practice, we are drawn back to key elements from Chapters 1 and 2. We think through how to make it experiential, how to engage different thinking and information-processing styles, and how to make it real for the participants.

We review the learning objectives to ensure that we are teaching them what the analysis indicated is important. By the end of this workshop, participants will be able to:

- Use an effective communications and delivery model to plan communications and select communication media

- Present data and information effectively

- Develop and deliver communications that positively influence others

We review our original thoughts about Sequence of Instruction (and Duration) and decide we are headed in the right direction. First, we have to get specific about how to carry out each method we have outlined. To illustrate, Table 3.1 expands on the example from Sample Worksheet 2.1 in Chapter 2.

TABLE 3.1 *Detailed Action Steps for Organizational-Level Communication Course*

TOPIC	METHOD	DURATION	ACTIONS
Welcome	Discuss	15 minutes	Discuss –Objectives –Ground Rules –Agenda
	Introductory Activity		Introductory Activity –Small Groups (3–5) –Answer: 　　Best communication experience 　　Worst communication experience –Large group debrief
Effective Communication	Mini-Lecture	30 minutes	Mini-Lecture –Joe's slides 12–16 –*Crucial Conversations*, Ch. 2
	Examples		Examples –Working on policies committee –Draw some from class
	Your own case		Your own case –Identify communication objective –Identify key barriers –Discuss with a partner –Large group debrief
Influencing Effectively	Mini-Lecture	30 minutes	Mini-Lecture –*Crucial Conversations*, Ch. 7 –*Leading with Questions*, Chs. 4 & 5
	Examples		Examples –Working on policies committee –Draw some from class
	Your own case		Your own case –Identify questions to use –Identify support you need –Discuss with a partner –Large group debrief

continues

TABLE 3.1 *Continued*

Topic	Method	Duration	Actions
Bringing It All Together	Prepare your case Practice with others	30 minutes	Prepare your case –Practice alone Practice with others –Groups of three (3 rotations) –Large group debrief
Next Steps	Reflection Share	15 minutes	Reflection –Answer questions in Participant Guide Share –Groups of three –Large group debrief –Thank participants

Completing this detailed level of development is important for a few reasons. First, by including more detail, you can begin to see if the time allocations are correct. The more times you do this, the more comfortable you will become with time allocation. Second, you begin to identify specific tasks you want the participants to accomplish. Third, this level of detail will help you build the slides and facilitator notes as well as the Participant Guide.

Next, we have to build the supporting PowerPoint deck with facilitator notes, as well as a Participant Guide and any other supporting materials we might need. This becomes an issue of finding adequate time to sit down, start developing the materials, and get someone to help you review the materials. In organizations that are a little busier or that don't provide you with a quiet office, you may find working from a more secluded location may be beneficial in brainstorming and creating content for a presentation. If you are looking for secluded locations, we can recommend a nice corner table at your local coffee house. Also, you can schedule a meeting room at your facility, preferably far away from your regular work area. If it's a nice day, find a patio! Content development takes time and definitely is worth the effort!

Here are a few things to remember about developing content:

- Your PowerPoint slides should add to the experience, not detract from it. See sidebar on PowerPointers for more tips.

- Write your facilitator/speaker notes as if someone who has never seen the content has been asked to facilitate. This will ensure that you get all the key points into your notes.

- The Participant Guide should not be a direct match to the slides. It should be a combination of what is on the slides as well as information in the facilitator notes.

POWERPOINTERS

We also want to offer a couple of pointers about PowerPoint. Surely you have seen some not-so-great presentations, so if you want to create a more impressive presentation, you may consider the following tidbits:

- *People tend to put a lot of information on their slides. Remember that according to Cliff Atkinson, author of* Beyond Bullet Points *(2011), if everything you're going to say is on the slide, one of you is redundant!*

  - *A good slide should have no more than three to five key points, including sub-bullets.*

  - *In order to make sub-bullets worthwhile, you should have at least two sub-bullets. Otherwise, don't use them!*

  - *We recommend that you do not go below 22-point font. Others might say 16-point, but we have found that keeping font size at 22-point or above helps keep you honest on the three to five key points suggestion.*

- *Never underestimate the power of a great photograph. For example, rather than putting the agenda on the slide, you could put a photograph of a map on the slide and talk about the agenda, as well as include it (the agenda) in the Participant Guide.*

- *When selecting a color scheme, use complementary or contrasting colors (for example, pick two colors on opposite sides of the color wheel).*

- *Avoid placing both red and green colors on the same slide because audience members who are color blind will be unable to differentiate between these.*

Figures 3.1 and 3.2 illustrate our take on what a slide with facilitator notes might look like as well as what the page might look like in the Participant Guide.

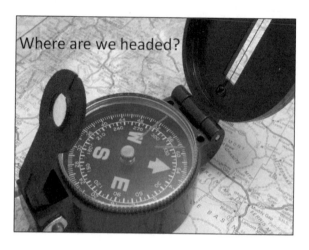

Say

Before we begin, I'd like to let you know where we are headed. If you'll turn to page 3 in your Participant Guide, you will find our learning objectives, agenda and ground rules for the day.

This module focuses on effective communication skills, including the ability to influence. You can see that you will get a chance to practice your own situation and we will discuss other examples as well.

Regarding our ground rules, let's agree that we will:
• Start and end on time.
• Respect differences.
• Participate fully.
• Turn electronic devices onto silent mode.
• Enjoy the process!

FIGURE 3.1

Sample organizational slide with speaker notes (displayed in Note View).

What you should notice about the slide and facilitator notes is:

• The photograph of the compass is a visual cue for direction.

• The title of the slide is consistent with the visual.

• The facilitator notes go into detail about the objectives, the agenda, and the ground rules.

Where are we headed?

Learning Objectives	By the end of this workshop, participants will be able to: • Use an effective communications and delivery model to plan communications and select communication media • Present data and information effectively • Develop and deliver communications that positively influence others

Agenda

Topic	Method	Duration
Welcome	• Discuss • Introductory Activity	15 minutes
Effective Communications	• Mini-Lecture • Examples • Your own case	30 minutes
Influencing Effectively	• Mini-Lecture • Examples • Your own case	30 minutes
Bringing It All Together	• Prepare your case • Practice with others • Receive feedback	30 minutes
Next Steps	• Reflection • Share	15 minutes

Ground Rules
- Start and end on time.
- Respect differences.
- Participate fully.
- Turn electronic devices onto silent mode.
- Enjoy the process!

Notes

_____

_____

_____

_____

_____

_____

FIGURE 3.2

Sample organizational Participant Guide page.

To help the participants, you should create a guide for them to use during the module. While the slide provides a visual cue of what is being discussed, the corresponding Participant Guide should provide the necessary detail. Notice that our Participant Guide example provides the detailed learning objectives, a high-level agenda, and the ground rules. Also, we left additional space for the participants to make any relevant notes.

Now that we have looked at an organizational-level example of slide, notes, and Participant Guide, we will look at a unit-level example (see Figures 3.3 and 3.4). Again, this example was developed by the authors specifically for this book. The unit-level example is about resuscitations for optimal results.

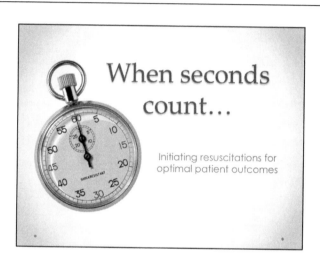

Say

Welcome, everyone! Today's topic will focus on the importance of timely recognition of cardiac arrests and initiating the emergency response system.

Go head and turn to the first page of your participant guide, and you'll find the learning objective, agenda, and ground rules. You'll see that we're going to spend some time discussing cardiac arrest situations, but the portion that most participants really enjoy is the end when we'll practice our new knowledge with a simulation.

Please review the ground rules, and let me know if you have any questions.

FIGURE 3.3

Sample unit slide with speaker notes (displayed in Note View).

The visual on this slide is perfect because the title of the module is "When seconds count…" The facilitator notes direct the participants to their Participant Guide for more specifics about the learning objectives, agenda, and ground rules. Does anyone see a pattern here? We do… what works for organization-level modules will work for unit-level modules. The concepts of the ADDIE model will work, regardless of what type of learning you are designing!

When seconds count...

Learning Objectives	By the end of this class, participants will be able to: • Recognize signs and symptoms of impending cardiac arrest • Describe the nurse's role in initiating a resuscitation for a cardiac arrest • Identify unit resources for managing a patient in cardiac arrest before the code team arrives

Agenda

Topic	Method	Duration
Welcome	• Discuss • Share Previous Experiences • Introductory Activity	15 minutes
Resuscitation Procedures	• Lecture • Vignettes	45 minutes
Resuscitation Practice	• Code Blue Simulation	45 minutes
Next Steps	• Reflection • Share	15 minutes

Ground Rules
- Start and end on time.
- Participate fully.
- Turn electronic devices onto silent mode.
- Enjoy the process!

Notes
_____
_____
_____
_____
_____
_____

FIGURE 3.4

Sample unit Participant Guide page.

I DON'T WANT TO LECTURE YOU, BUT...

...some presentations can be dull and dry. Here are some ways you can keep your lecture component engaging and lively:

- *Your presentation shouldn't be just you speaking. Invite participation by asking questions or by having participants discuss something and report back to the larger group.*

- *Ask open-ended questions to get the discussion going. Use closed questions (yes/no) very sparingly, because they close down a discussion.*

- *If appropriate, involve activity; allow everyone to get up and move around at some point.*

- *Any "lecture" should be 20 minutes long or less. At that point, engage participants in an activity that is related to the content you just shared.*

- *Consider using videos where appropriate. When Alvin teaches other nurses about different types of seizures, he uses video to show the unique aspects of each type of seizure. A picture is still worth a thousand words!*

- *Use hands-on equipment when it makes sense. For example, would you teach someone about fire safety and not include a fire extinguisher?*

Centralized AND Decentralized Programs

The best onboarding program includes both centralized and decentralized aspects. That said, many of you may work for organizations in which you are responsible for the organization- and unit-level programs, or you may be responsible for one or the other. Best practices would suggest that at an organizational level, you want to cover topics such as:

- Organizational mission, vision, and values

- Organizational culture—formal and informal

- Key HR guidelines and policies

- Facility tour

- Safety training

The benefits of covering these topics at an organizational level are tremendous. Your nurses will be meeting nurses from other units, as well as other key personnel. This helps build an organizational-level support system for them. Additionally, it's good to get the interdisciplinary insights about the organization. In some organizations, this type of orientation will allow them to meet (or see via video) key executives in the organization.

At the unit level, you will want to cover things that are specific to your unit. These might include:

- Unit mission and vision (if available) along with outcomes data or performance measures

- Unit culture—formal and informal

- Unit-specific guidelines, policies, and procedures

- Unit tour

- Patient and family demographics

Most of you don't need us to point out the benefits of unit-level onboarding, but we will highlight a few for you. At the unit level, the culture might have a slightly different spin than the organizational level, and it's important for your new nurses to understand these nuances. Also, your new nurses may never have worked with the types of patients you see on your floor, so this gives you an opportunity to help them understand those differences as well.

A huge part of onboarding is helping your orientees understand the organizational and unit cultures. As we all know, culture really has two elements—the formal and informal aspects. Culture is something that is difficult to teach; however, here are a few ideas:

- Formal aspects of the culture should be discussed early and often. These aspects include organizational and unit-level mission and vision as well as organizational values and social responsibility commitments.

- If you have people in a cohort, give them opportunities to meet and discuss what they have learned about the culture. These discussions probably will be focused on informal aspects of the culture.

- Preceptors should be prepared to answer questions about formal and informal culture in addition to questions about procedures, processes, and policies.

- Give orientees a chance in one-on-one situations to ask any question they wish. You can even provide suggestions of questions they might want answered in order to make them comfortable with asking these questions.

Nurse Residency Programs

Nurse residency programs (e.g., the University HealthSystem Consortium/American Association of Colleges of Nursing [UHC/AACN] Nurse Residency Program or the Versant Residency Programs) could be a great asset to you and your organization. These programs are primarily known for their ability to assist new graduate RNs in being successful during their first year in the workplace. However, these programs are being modified and expanded to include RNs who have moved to new specialties as well. By providing support and professional development activities for new employees, these programs have demonstrated a high degree of efficacy in reducing turnover and increasing satisfaction. From a design and implementation perspective, a benefit of these programs is the amount of guidance provided to you since a program structure is already outlined. These programs have a variety of curriculum pathways, evaluation surveys, course content, and evidence-based practice materials already created. For more information on these programs, check out their websites (https://www.uhc.edu/16807.htm and https://www.versant.org/).

Anatomy of a Unit's Onboarding Program

By this point in the book, we've covered a lot of different principles, principals, methods, programs, considerations, etc. Hopefully, by now you have more of an idea of how to evaluate the onboarding program you currently have and design, develop, and implement the one that you need. This final portion of the development/implementation part of the book is devoted to helping unit-based educators construct an effective onboarding program at the unit level. If you're more of a visual learner and want to see where we're heading, jump to the end and check out Figure 3.5 to see where these components fit into the orientee's overall experience.

Selecting Preceptors

Selecting a preceptor (or multiple preceptors) for a new employee can certainly be a bit stressful because this decision will determine who his/her most significant teacher will be during the learning experience. There are many factors that influence selection of preceptors, and these could be simplified to include both the availability of preceptors as well as the professional development needs of nurses on the unit.

Availability issues could include:

- Lack of available preceptors if you are orienting a large number of orientees at one time

- Scheduling conflicts between orientee requests or classes and those of the preceptors

- Mismatch between the numbers of hours worked per week (for example, an orientee may be hired for full-time employment while the ideal preceptor works only part-time)

Professional development issues could include:

- Clinical advancement, because some organizations require precepting as a prerequisite

- The manager's request for the use of a particular preceptor based on recommendations from performance management

- Inexperience of the preceptor (for example, some newer preceptors may be intimidated by having an orientee who has many years of experience in another area, or if a unit comprises primarily newer staff, it may be difficult to find a nurse with enough experience to serve as a preceptor)

There are also some situations in which both availability and professional development needs may play a role in the selection of a preceptor (some nurses who served as preceptors may become charge nurses and therefore unable to serve in this dual role). In addition to these, we're sure you could think of several other problems in selecting ideal preceptors for your new staff. What follows are some key points we've identified that are important to consider when selecting preceptors.

From a practical perspective, you always want to select your preceptors as early as possible in the orientation/onboarding process. This allows you to *ask* the preceptor if they're able and willing to serve in this role rather than *telling* them due to last-minute planning.

TIP

Although each preceptor will have a different preference, we recommend asking the preceptor in person rather than through email or a phone call. Not everyone loves precepting, so while they may offer to do it, speaking with them in person allows you to assess any nonverbal cues that may assist you in providing the optimal amount of support for your preceptors.

Team vs. Individual Preceptors

Based on the unique combination of preceptor availability and professional development needs in your organization, you may be able to assign multiple (team) preceptors versus single (individual) preceptors to an orientee. There are pros and cons to both of these approaches, which we outline in Table 3.2.

TABLE 3.2 *Comparison of Team and Individual Preceptor Structures*

	TEAM		INDIVIDUAL	
	PROS	**CONS**	**PROS**	**CONS**
Scheduling	Allows the use of part-time preceptors	Requires availability of many preceptors	Easy to develop	May pose many conflicts with orientee requests and classes
Experience	Able to see multiple "ways of doing it"	Some items may fall through the cracks	Consistency in relationship (able to ensure progress)	Only exposed to one "way of doing it"
Preceptor Satisfaction	No single preceptor carries the full weight of teaching	Potential for conflict on team	Able to develop very strong relationship with orientee	No teaching breaks during orientation

Without knowing the unique situation in your organization, we recommend the team precepting approach. As long as you have enough preceptors to form teams, the benefits of this approach in overcoming the barriers of availability and professional development needs are substantial. Teams could comprise two to four preceptors (depending on hours worked per week, experience level, etc.), and ideally, the teams should remain exclusive and consistent (that is, preceptors are only on one team at a time, and they do not switch to another team with the next orientee).

Additionally, team precepting may actually enhance professional development of some preceptors because newer preceptors can be placed on a team with more experienced preceptors. This can decrease the stress of newer preceptors (since they are not responsible for teaching the orientees everything they need to know), while providing a safe environment for receiving feedback (experienced preceptors can observe an orientee's performance and relay information to newer preceptors).

Communication and Learning/Teaching Styles

Check out the potential preceptors' MBTI or VARK results. Most people naturally teach in the same style they learn, so if you can match preceptors and orientees based on similarities, this may prove beneficial.

If the preceptor and orientee cannot be matched based on similar styles (due to a limited preceptor pool or a less-common style), you should anticipate that the preceptor might need more assistance or guidance in effective teaching strategies. Even experienced preceptors may encounter situations in which they are stumped regarding how to appropriately convey a concept. This could be due to a lack of training and development in effective and varied teaching strategies. Consider holding preceptor workshops for new *and* experienced preceptors to support their development.

PRECEPTOR WORKSHOPS

If you think your preceptors could benefit from some training and development of their own, you might want to hold a workshop or inservice for them. Here are some topics you could cover that preceptors are likely to find valuable:

- *Diverse learning styles (for example, discuss the VARK theory and strategies for precepting an orientee whose preferred learning style is different from the preceptor's)*
- *Conflict management*
- *Giving and receiving feedback*
- *How to debrief an orientee following a traumatic event*
- *Evaluating competency*

Does the Preceptor Want to Precept?

We mentioned earlier the importance of *asking* preceptors if they're willing and able to precept rather than *telling* them they have to. But what if the preceptor responds with a big "No!" when you ask her?

First, explore *why* she is refusing to precept. Has she recently had a bad experience with an orientee? Is she serving as a primary nurse for a patient and doesn't want to take different patients? Are there personal reasons (for example, an ill family member or a divorce) that the preceptor worries will influence her ability to give precepting her full attention? Or does she simply hate precepting? Determining the cause of her refusal will help you find a solution, if possible.

Take for an example the preceptor who had a bad experience or the one who hates precepting. Perhaps his problems arise from inadequate development of his precepting skills. Consider placing him in a preceptor development course or working with him one-on-one to give him better strategies for working with orientees. You could also speak with his manager to see if this is a nurse who should not be precepting; if so, find ways for him to contribute to the unit through other leadership activities.

Similarly, if a preceptor has significant problems in her personal life, it is probably best to allow a break from precepting. If paired with an orientee, the preceptor may feel extremely dissatisfied with her work, which could influence the quality of learning the orientee achieves. You should make sure the preceptor's manager is aware of her inability to serve in this role since this responsibility is likely in the employee's job description. However, it is important to be respectful of the preceptor's situation, and you can maintain a healthy relationship with the preceptor by discussing your desire to leverage her precepting capabilities once she feels well enough to do so again.

Finally, for the preceptor who is serving as a primary nurse, you must weigh the pros and cons of optimal preceptor selection and optimal nurse-patient relationships. This is likely a decision that needs to be made among leadership at the unit/department level, as it will influence both the quality of nurses completing orientation as well as the quality of care received by the individual patient who has a primary nurse. If a compromise could be made (e.g., the primary nurse serves as a preceptor but is able to be in close proximity to the selected patient almost every shift), that may be worth exploring.

Regardless of why someone doesn't want to precept, if you are unable to change her attitude, we recommend not using her to precept, if possible. People who hate what they're doing probably aren't going to be good at it. The orientee may receive a better learning experience from a less experienced preceptor who loves doing it, rather than a more experienced preceptor who is burned out.

RED FLAGS OF A BURNED-OUT PRECEPTOR

Watch for the following signs that your preceptors may be burned out or unfocused:

- *When asked if willing to precept, he/she hesitates or even provides nonverbal communication of disinterest (for example, a sigh or an eye roll).*
- *When working with an orientee, the preceptor is found socializing or reading a book rather than observing and teaching the orientee.*
- *The preceptor frequently calls in sick or makes last-minute schedule changes on days when he/she is assigned to have an orientee.*
- *When the orientee performs a task incorrectly, the preceptor quickly resorts to verbal or physical abuse rather than constructive feedback.*
- *The preceptor is observed talking with colleagues about being "forced to precept" or "never being able to take care of patients by myself."*
- *Or very simply, the preceptor asks you for a break.*

Motivating Preceptors

On a more positive note, we want to discuss some ways you can motivate your nurses to serve as preceptors. It's not an easy task, so providing external motivators and facilitating internal motivators may be beneficial in maintaining a healthy work environment. Table 3.3 has some ideas to get you thinking.

TABLE 3.3 *Preceptor Motivators*

External Rewards	• Hold focus groups or send out surveys to determine desirable external rewards
	• Monetary incentives (e.g., differentials while precepting, bonuses upon orientee completion)
	• Organize appreciation events (e.g., schedule a dinner event off campus and invite key administrators to attend the event, too)
Internal Rewards	• Help preceptors realize the contribution they are making to the next generation of nurses (e.g., point out to them how the high-functioning nurses on the unit were previously orientees of theirs)
	• Provide preceptor development opportunities to make the experience more enjoyable
	• Encourage orientees to write thank-you notes to preceptors upon completion of orientation

Introduction to Unit/Department

Once you've selected your preceptors, given your new employees their schedules, and ensured completion of central (organizational) orientation requirements, the orientees are ready to come to the unit! Before immediately placing them with their preceptors, you'll want to welcome them to the unit/department with an initial tour and overview. Just as the organization at-large has unique policies, procedures, guidelines, cultural nuances, and many new faces, so does the unit. If you place orientees with a preceptor and a patient assignment on the first day on the unit, orientees will be lacking fundamental knowledge to be successful (for example, how to clock-in, where to retrieve medications, and maybe even where to find a bathroom). Scheduling even a few hours to cover housekeeping and cultural issues will significantly enhance the orientee's experience.

Each unit will be unique in what should be covered, but here's what Alvin tells his new hires regarding what needs to be addressed: "The purpose of today's introduction to the unit is so that when you are with your preceptor tomorrow, you: (a) know where to go and how to get there and (b) have everything you need to focus entirely on your patient assignment rather than worrying about getting lost or not having access to something important." You can see why the actual components could be quite unique to each unit. For an example agenda, check out Table 3.4.

TABLE 3.4 *Example Agenda for an Introduction to the Unit/Department*

Getting Around	Provide walking tour of unit/department, and be sure to include:
	• Break rooms and meeting rooms
	• Bathrooms
	• Lockers/showers
	• Manager, educators, and other administrative offices
	• Supply closets
	• Time clock
	• Where to receive assignment/report at beginning of shift
	• Fire extinguishers*
	• Gas shut-off valves*
	• Emergency exits and evacuation plan*
	Ensure access to secured locations and services (for example, medication administration equipment, electronic documentation systems, supply closets, alternative entry/exit doors, etc.).
Socialization	Introduce new employee to the following people:
	• Manager
	• Educator
	• Preceptor
	• During walking tour, introduce to various other staff along the way
	• Administrative personnel (for example, payroll specialist)
	Consider taking photographs of new employees and having them write brief bios to post for current staff.

continues

TABLE 3.4 *Continued*

Documentation	Complete, sign, and file:
	• Department orientation form* (typically, a checklist verifying discussion of policies/procedures along with various expectations of manager and employee)
	• Equipment agreements (for example, pagers or keys), if loaning equipment from the unit
	• Unit-specific honesty, integrity, or HIPAA forms
Expectations	Discuss and/or set the following standards with new employees:
	• Unit-specific policies, procedures, and/or guidelines
	• Unspoken or tacit rules (for example, in which refrigerator should they place their lunchbox)
	• Requirements for completing orientation (target behaviors, learning activities, etc.)

Those items noted with an asterisk may be a requirement of a regulatory body, depending on your particular organization. Refer to Chapter 7 or your specific regulatory body's requirements.

We recommend creating a checklist of the agenda you develop for your unit and keeping a signed copy of completion in the orientee's record. Doing that may help to demonstrate compliance with regulatory requirements.

> **TIP**
>
> Additionally, you may want to consider creating and maintaining a spreadsheet or checklist of your own that will ensure all necessary requirements and components of starting a new employee are covered. It can become quite overwhelming to verify receipt or completion of necessary paperwork, and keeping a spreadsheet will help you stay organized.

Time With Patients

Once an orientee has completed organizational orientation and received an introduction to the unit/department, he/she is finally ready to begin his/her precepted experiences and care for patients. Getting to this point may feel like an eternity for the new employee, especially if he/she is a new graduate nurse. This time (and especially the first day) is fairly exciting for most orientees, as it's the point where the rubber meets the road, so to speak. Although the preceptor and orientee begin to take the reins here, the educator and manager remain extremely important in this transition period.

We recommend checking in frequently during the orientee's first few days of taking care of patients to provide support to the orientee and preceptor, ensure the orientee has access to all necessary systems and equipment, and look for any red flags that may immediately surface. Whatever it is that may surface, **do not wait** to address the situation. Even if the situation may work itself out, intervening early is always beneficial because it not only demonstrates support for the preceptor and orientee but also prevents wasting time if the situation needs escalation to more formal interventions.

THE TOP RED FLAGS TO WATCH FOR IN THE FIRST FEW DAYS

During those first few days, be observant, and if you see any of the following red flags, consider quickly intervening:

- *Gross incompetence, carelessness, or negligence in the particular setting*
- *Orientee's verbalization of feeling he/she made a terrible decision to accept this job*
- *Atypical display of emotions such as crying or becoming completely silent*
- *Overconfidence displayed by the orientee frequently stating "I know that" or attempting to perform procedures without supervision*
- *Calling in sick or not reporting in for an assigned shift*
- *Taking frequent breaks*

Educators and managers can assist preceptors and charge nurses in selecting patient assignments that provide new learning opportunities while also reinforcing previously acquired knowledge. Due to the complexity of the healthcare environment and patient presentations, the learning trajectory is rarely linear. Preceptors may have to reinforce some concepts on more than one occasion. For concerns that arise, you may want to check out Chapter 5 for more detailed information on working with different types of orientees.

Other Learning Experiences

Although the majority of learning will occur while actually spending time with patients, other unit-based activities can be developed and implemented to augment patient care experiences. These could be taught by educators, expert or clinically advanced nurses, and even nurse practitioners or physicians. Certain limitations, typically financial, will always be present when augmenting patient care with these additional learning opportunities; however, well-designed activities are quite beneficial and a key component of most great orientation programs.

Classroom

Unit-specific didactic classes can be very useful for orientees, especially if they are conducted early in the orientation experience. We recommend providing only one or two classes per week because it is also important to have the opportunity to apply the information gained in class to the clinical setting. Beneficial topics for classroom content can be determined through speaking with key stakeholders, but general ideas include:

- Most commonly seen diagnoses or procedures

- Difficult, complex, or confusing skills performed on the unit

- Time-sensitive skills that should be explained before they are experienced in a clinical setting (for example, resuscitation procedures)

- Situations that are emotionally challenging or difficult to discuss in the clinical environment

- Processes that preceptors may not have sufficient time to thoroughly discuss during a clinical shift

TIP

Consider partnering with other units to organize classes. This fosters interdepartmental relationships and offers orientees new insights or different perspectives on caring for patients. Additionally, it prevents reinventing the wheel if another department already has a well-designed class in place.

Skills Lab

Similar to the classroom setting, a skills lab provides orientees with the opportunity to learn and practice psychomotor skills without the fear of harming patients. You may want to include skills lab sessions as a part of classroom instruction (this helps to break up the didactic content and keep learners engaged). You don't need a physical room dedicated as a skills lab to provide excellent learning opportunities for new employees. You could find an empty patient room or bring supplies to a conference room or classroom. Orientees can benefit from things as simple as operating a peripheral intravenous catheter's safety device, drawing up unusual medications, preparing a drainage system for a chest tube, or even applying a 12-lead electrocardiogram to a female manikin.

Simulation

Simulation is becoming a big focus in healthcare education, both in academic and service settings. The opportunity to practice interdisciplinary teamwork, especially in rare or life-threatening situations, is a key benefit of simulation, and research is beginning to validate these benefits. Including simulation to practice skills such as resuscitation or end-of-life care can be invaluable for orientees.

Conclusion

This is probably a lot to take in, especially if you have no experience in developing an entire orientation program. While the previous content has focused specifically on developing individual chunks of an orientation/onboarding program, the following Figure 3.5 provides a generic timeline for moving an orientee from accepting a job offer to independent practice.

Before 1st Day

- Employee contacted by manager and educator (e.g., a phone call
- Access requested for necessary systems & applications (e.g., electronic documentation, medication dispensing equipment, etc.)
- Necessary classes are scheduled, or the employee is registered for standing classes
- Orientation & onboarding schedule is sent to new employee

Organizational Orientation

- Manager and/or educator welcome new employee in-person
- Employee attends Organization/Central orientation (mission/vision, values, organizational policies/procedures, cultural overiew)
- Employee registers for benefits & completes other HR forms (e.g., income tax forms)
- Tour facility & meet key executives
- Complete educational orientation actvities required of all employees (e.g., safety training, infection control)

Unit/Department Orientation

- Manager and/or educator welcome new employee in-person
- Tour unit & meet key personnel (including preceptor, if possible)
- Review of unit policies/procedures/guidelines
- Discuss expectations of unit/department onboarding

Unit/Department Onboarding

- New employee completes required education activites (classes, online modules, shadow experiences, etc.)
- New employee provides care for patients under preceptor supervision
- Regular meetings scheduled with the orientee, preceptor, educator, and manager

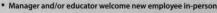

FIGURE 3.5

Timeline for orientation & onboarding progression of a new employee.

Questions for Reflection and Discussion

1. What challenges do you see in assembling and utilizing effective preceptors? What rewards could you easily facilitate for your preceptors?

2. What additional components should be added to the unit introduction for your own unit/department?

3. What role could you see classes, skills labs, and/or simulations playing in your orientation program?

KEY TAKEAWAYS

- *Set aside adequate time to developing educational content.*
- *Use the worksheet provided to help you develop specific modules for your program.*
- *Consider using a variety of teaching strategies that involve external resources, internal resources from other departments, and diverse educational media.*
- *Carefully select and adequately prepare preceptors for each new orientee as this will be the orientee's most significant teacher.*
- *From formal organizational culture to informal unit-based culture and everything in between, onboarding a new hire takes a large amount of planning and effort (but it's worth it).*

References

Atkinson, C. (2011). *Beyond bullet points* (3rd ed.). Redmond, WA: Microsoft Press.

CHAPTER 4

Evaluating an Individual's Competency

Introduction

Having read this far in this book, you either already have a good idea of what it takes to build an orientation program, or you may already have an orientation program running (which may or may not be easily changed). Regardless, determining an individual's competency is the most pivotal moment during the orientation experience. This is the point where the new employee, preceptor, and other stakeholders decide if the individual is ready to practice independently. We identify this as the most pivotal moment due to the potential for harming patients if a nurse is identified as competent in his/her setting, when in fact, he/she may not be.

This chapter will explore various methods for assessing competency and the role of key stakeholders in the determination of competency. Your particular organization or unit/department will have to determine where to set the bar for what competency looks like, given your specific patient population. However, the tools for evaluating competency are universal; the goals you set or outcomes you hope to see upon evaluation will vary.

Time-Based vs. Competency-Based Programs

You need to determine whether you will use a time-based or a competency-based approach to orientation and onboarding. The camp to which you subscribe will be a fundamental decision in the design of your orientation program, as it will influence stakeholder expectations, guide their actions, and assist you in predicting the allocation of an organization's resources.

- **Time-based programs** have a standard or predetermined length of orientation, and those orientees who are not meeting desired behaviors are given a longer period of orientation.

- **Competency-based programs** have a length of orientation that varies based on the individual and the learning opportunities he/she receives.

Alvin's experience in learning how other organizations implement orientation is that most of them are time-based. Very few organizations have a competency-based orientation program in which orientation ends at the point in which desired behaviors are achieved. Figure 4.1 provides a visual representation of these two approaches.

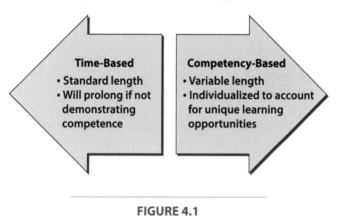

FIGURE 4.1

Approaches to orientation length.

We believe a competency-based approach is ideal because it allows for individualization of the orientation experience, which should result in more effective learning and, hypothetically, a more competent nurse. However, traditional time-based orientation programs may be difficult to change. Hopefully, we can convince you of the benefits of a competency-based approach.

What Is Competency?

Competency can be defined and described in a number of ways, but we propose the following simple definition. *Competency* is the ability to perform the job tasks and duties for which one was hired. We believe this definition's simplicity allows it to be applied to multiple organizations and settings. This definition also means that when *you* are defining competency in your area, you will need to keep a copy of the job description on hand. Assessing competency can be approached through many mechanisms, and we have highlighted several of them in this chapter through exploration of the following considerations:

- Distinguishing between competence and confidence

- Nurturing critical thinking and interpersonal skills

- Recognizing the Novice to Expert continuum (Benner, 1982, 2004)

- Using learning domains (cognitive, psychomotor, and affective) to assess and teach

Understanding Competence vs. Confidence

As you evaluate your orientees, you must keep in mind the difference between competence and confidence. Although this may seem rather simple at first, distinguishing between the two becomes important in the event a new employee perceives his/her competence differently than the perception of others. For purposes of this discussion, we assume *competence* is the degree to which someone is able to practice nursing safely under various conditions, as measured by objective tools and/or other healthcare providers' observations. Conversely, *confidence* will be defined as the self-assessed (perceived) degree to which someone is able to practice nursing safely under various conditions.

We define these in this way due to the frequency with which these words are used among practicing clinicians and educators alike. However, more accurate labels would be *subjective (self) competence* (instead of confidence) and *objective competence* (instead of competence). This labeling recognizes the value of the individual in assessing competence, an important activity for all stakeholders.

But we'll go back to using *competence* and *confidence* because these terms may be more commonly used in the practice setting. Furthermore, for purposes of simplicity, we want to assume that both competence and confidence could be either high or low (knowing full well that a very large continuum could be constructed to indicate where someone falls on the actual scale). Using high and low as values, Table 4.1 highlights the four possible combinations of these two variables (competence and confidence) and what to expect in an orientee.

TABLE 4.1 *Comparisons of Various Combinations of Competence and Confidence*

		COMPETENCE (OBJECTIVE)	
		HIGH	LOW
CONFIDENCE (SUBJECTIVE)	HIGH	Demonstrates that both the individual and others agree that competence has been achieved. The orientee is ready to practice independently. Action: Complete orientation.	The orientee's perception of his/her performance is greater than that of others' perceptions. This could be problematic in the event an orientee is not receptive to feedback. Action: Provide open and honest feedback to orientee. Ensure all stakeholders understand expectations for demonstrating competency. Encourage reflection on performance.
	LOW	The orientee is practicing safely but doubts his/her own abilities. This could be problematic if the fear or anxiety is so great that errors occur due to this emotional distress. Action: Focus on growth, reaffirm strengths, and highlight performance so far.	Demonstrates that both the individual and others agree that competence has not been achieved. The orientee is either (a) still actively learning or (b) unfortunately working in an environment that may not be a good fit for his/her skill level and interests. Action: Continue orientation if actively learning. Consider transfer or termination if environment is not a good fit.

The ideal situations would occur when the degree of both confidence and competence are identical (both high or both low). Those situations represent expected positions in the learning trajectory. However, if the confidence and competence levels do not match, you might have some challenges. For example, if competence is high and confidence is low, patient safety is not of paramount concern but the employee's satisfaction with his/her job or role is. This may be a normal developmental phase for many new graduate nurses (for more information, check out the story of Moldable Molly in Chapter 5). The least desirable situation occurs when confidence is high but competence is low. An orientee experiencing this situation will require extra attention from preceptors and other stakeholders to become successful.

Competence and confidence, while both desired in practice and frequently interchanged in casual conversation, are two very different concepts. Being able to differentiate between the two, especially when there is a need for improvement, will be key in developing appropriate interventions to help the orientee.

Nurturing Critical-Thinking and Interpersonal Skills

An aspect of nursing that creates ambiguity in assessing competence is the need for orientees to possess and continue to develop critical-thinking and interpersonal skills. Like other healthcare fields, complex situations are almost a guarantee due to an ever-changing environment and nurse-client relationship. If nursing were limited to caring for value-free machines, the issue of assessing competence would be much simpler (which is actually the case when evaluating skills performed in a laboratory or simulated setting). However, the real world is much more complex and requires a balance of hands-on *critical-thinking* and *interpersonal* skills.

For example, inserting a urinary catheter into a manikin involves following a set of structured steps. However, inserting a urinary catheter into an irritable, febrile infant who presents to an outpatient clinic accompanied by four older siblings who want to "help" is a bit more difficult. It is this discrepancy between academia and practice that can make interventions and evaluation methods developed in the academic setting difficult to apply to the service setting.

Although we would love to provide you with a magic wand to help with teaching and assessing these critical-thinking and interpersonal skills, we only are able to emphasize that these are competencies that must be acquired before being able to practice safely. We don't have the space to define and describe these terms along with potential methods of evaluation, but there are critical thinking measurement tools that exist (for example, Health Sciences Reasoning Test [Insight Assessment, 2013]) and that can be created (for example, situational judgment tests).

EXAMPLE QUESTION FROM A SITUATIONAL JUDGMENT TEST

You are currently caring for a six-patient assignment (maximum allowed per policy) on a busy surgical ward. One of your colleagues becomes sick and has to leave. You are told that you must take three of your colleague's patients. On a scale of 1–5, how appropriate are each of the following actions?

   a. Refusing to take report on the additional patients
   b. Calling the charge nurse or manager for assistance
   c. Delegating nursing tasks (such as medication administration) to the unlicensed assistive personnel
   d. Reprioritizing your tasks to accommodate the increased workload
   e. Asking the patient's family members to help with activities of daily living
   f. Delaying documentation in the patients' records until additional help arrives

Critical-thinking and interpersonal skills can be difficult to evaluate objectively because each nurse-client relationship will exist in differing situations. However, they are necessary skills, and we encourage you to delay an orientee's completion of orientation if you think his/her capacity for these skills is substandard. The important part is assisting the orientee to develop in this area. Here are some examples that may get you started in helping your orientee:

- Administer case studies that focus on critical-thinking assessment (many books have been published to provide premade scenarios).

- Create simulated scenarios to evaluate and teach desired skills (these could involve as much or as little technology and simulators as you want).

- Focus on strengthening emotional intelligence.

- Converse with orientee and explore thought process through "What if...?" questions (for example, What if the patient would have actually had no breath sounds on the right...what would you have done then? What if the patient doesn't speak English? What if you were to get an unexpected admission? What if the catheter became clogged?).

CRITICAL-THINKING CASE STUDIES

There are many books available with premade critical-thinking case studies for various patient care environments. Some case studies are even available for free with a quick search in your favorite Internet search engine. Here is a brief list of books you might want to check out:

- *Melander, S. D. (2004). Case Studies in Critical Care Nursing: A Guide for Application and Review (3rd ed.). Saunders.*

- *Harding, M. M., Snyder, J. S., Preusser, B. A. (2012). Winningham's Critical Thinking Cases in Nursing: Medical-Surgical, Pediatric, Maternity, and Psychiatric. St. Louis, MO: Mosby.*

- *Anker, G. M. (2011). Delmar's Case Study Series: Medical-Surgical Nursing (2nd ed.). Clifton Park, NY: Delmar.*

- *Lunney, M. (2009). Critical Thinking to Achieve Positive Health Outcomes: Nursing Case Studies and Analyses (2nd ed.). Ames, IA: Wiley Blackwell.*

LEARNING MORE ABOUT EMOTIONAL INTELLIGENCE

Emotional Intelligence (EI) comprises four pillars: Self-Awareness, Self-Management, Social Awareness, and Relationship Management (Goleman, 2006). Over the past few years, much focus has been placed on researching the connection between effective nursing practices and Emotional Intelligence. If you wish to learn more about EI, check first with your Human Resources department or Training and Development department. They might have coursework or reading materials available for you.

continues

If you would like to learn more about EI in the context of nursing, here are a few relevant articles that may be of help:

- *Akerjordet, K., & Severinsson, E. (2007). Emotional intelligence: A review of the literature with a specific focus on empirical and epistemological perspectives.* Journal of Clinical Nursing, 16(8), 1405-1416.
- *Freshwater, D., & Stickley, T. (2004). The heart of the art: Emotional intelligence in nurse education.* Nursing Inquiry, 11(2), 91-98.
- *McQueen, A. C. H. (2004). Emotional intelligence in nursing work.* Journal of Advanced Nursing, 47(1), 101-108.

For critical thinking, more specifically, it is probably quite a rare occurrence that an orientee has a significant problem with critical thinking if he/she were able to successfully complete his/her academic preparation and pass the licensure exam. Nevertheless, it is possible, so we have outlined an approach to evaluating and managing this possibility. This approach (the OPQRST process) is explained in Table 4.2.

TABLE 4.2 *OPQRST Process for Approaching Struggles with Critical Thinking*

	DESCRIPTION	RATIONALE
Objectivity	Explore objective accounts of concerning behaviors	Presuming what the orientee is thinking before observing what he or she is doing could lead to inaccurate conclusions
Patterns	Look for a pattern or theme that occurs across multiple scenarios	Assists with discovering the underlying problem while also considering the potential for situation-dependent factors
Qualify & Quantify	Qualify and/or quantify the impact these patterns could have on patient care	Measuring impact will help you determine the severity of the problem but will also provide an answer to the "So what?" question if the orientee asks
Reframe & Share	Help the orientee look at the situation from a different perspective (reframe) by sharing the emerging pattern or theme with the orientee	Raises the orientee's awareness of the problem (although, he/she likely is aware of the problem) and helps explore why the orientee proceeded the way he/she did

	DESCRIPTION	RATIONALE
Trial	Try alternative methods for approaching situations	Helps the orientee discover that often there is more than one way to approach a situation, and can help him/her begin to make appropriate distinctions

Recognizing the Novice to Expert Continuum

Patricia Benner's "From Novice to Expert" article published in 1982 was monumental in describing nursing skill levels, and the model helps inform another aspect of competency—the idea that a new nurse cannot be expected to know *everything* at the beginning of his or her career. Benner's model outlines five major stages of skill acquisition: novice, advanced beginner, competent, proficient, and expert. You can read brief descriptions of these stages in Table 4.3.

TABLE 4.3 *Patricia Benner's "From Novice to Expert" Model*

STAGE	DESCRIPTION
Novice	• Nonexperienced beginners • Rule-based, context-free decision-making • First Year of Education
Advanced Beginner	• Marginally acceptable performance • Beginning to recognize patterns from experiences • New Graduate
Competent	• Actions are viewed in light of long-term plans • Well-organized and deliberate • 1 to 2 Years in Practice
Proficient	• Situations perceived as a "whole" • Decision-making becomes automatic • A Transitional Stage on the Way to Expertise
Expert	• Intuitively understands the entire situation • Has trouble articulating what is known due to the depth with which it is known • Practical Wisdom

Source: Benner, 1982, 2004

Competence, as defined by Benner, is different than the definition of competency we are discussing in this chapter. Benner (1982) noted the stage of "Competent" was not achieved until one had been a nurse for 2 to 3 years (hopefully you won't have a new employee in orientation for that long!). For purposes of completing onboarding, you likely are looking for a nurse who has achieved the status of "Advanced Beginner." Keeping Benner's framework in mind will help you appreciate the development through which new nurses grow and may prevent you from setting expectations that are too high for new employees.

Using Domains of Learning to Assess and Teach

At this point in the book, we hope you have begun to appreciate the complexity of nursing orientation and onboarding as well as the varied approaches necessary to ensure individual competency. One simple structured method of performing this orientation and onboarding is to organize competency requirements into their respective domains of learning (cognitive, psychomotor, and affective). We label this as a simple structure because the learning domains lend themselves to evaluation using three simple questions:

- **Cognitive**—Has the orientee demonstrated he/she knows a sufficient amount to safely care for patients?

- **Psychomotor**—Has the orientee successfully performed skills that demonstrate the ability to safely care for patients?

- **Affective**—Are the orientee's words and actions congruent with the values and beliefs of both the organization and the patient population?

Cognitive Knowledge

Cognitive knowledge involves the ability to think, remember, reason, and problem-solve using one's mental capacities (for example, recognizing a decompensating patient or calculating a medication dose). Measurement of cognitive knowledge acquisition can be done through verbal or written methods but should answer the question, "Has the orientee demonstrated he/she knows a sufficient amount to care safely for patients?"

Cognitive teaching (and learning) can be facilitated through the following mechanisms:

- Instructor-led classes
- Online modules
- Assigned readings
- Observation of experienced nurses in the clinical setting

Cognitive learning can be measured through the following methods (among others):

- Tests and quizzes
- Question-and-answer discussion
- Documentation review
- Case studies

Psychomotor Skills

Psychomotor skills include the hands-on performance of tasks (for example, obtaining vital signs or inserting a feeding tube). Measurement of psychomotor skills is done by observation of the skill. Assessment should answer the question: "Has the orientee successfully performed skills that demonstrate the ability to care safely for patients?"

Psychomotor skill teaching (and learning) can be facilitated through the following mechanisms:

- Observation of experienced nurses in the clinical setting
- Simulation scenarios or skills laboratories
- Online modules (especially if they contain pictures and/or videos)

You are a little more limited in the number of options available for measuring psychomotor skill acquisition:

- Direct observation of skill
- Achievement of desired outcome (for example, verifying correct placement of feeding tube even though you did not observe the tube being placed)

Affective Thoughts and Behaviors

Affective knowledge is a person's integration of values, beliefs, and motivation. Facilitating, teaching, and evaluating in the affective domain is probably the most difficult of the three. Appropriate evaluation will answer the question, "Are the orientee's words and actions congruent with the values and beliefs of the organization, the employee, and the patient population?"

The affective domain is unique in that the methods for teaching also serve as the methods for evaluation. Some methods may include:

- Case studies

- Group discussion

- Guided reflection

EVALUATING AFFECTIVE THOUGHTS AND BEHAVIORS

Evaluating affective thoughts and behaviors is suited to the three methods of case studies, group discussions, and guided reflection. The nice thing about that is you can use the same example and apply it to all three methods.

Here is a scenario that you could use—a 3-week-old infant has been brought to the ER with a potential for having been abused by the mother's boyfriend. Both the mother and the boyfriend brought the baby into the ER and want to be present with the child. Hospital policy does not restrict visitation until an arrest has been made. You are the nurse caring for the child.

- *How would you handle this situation?*
- *What do you anticipate your conversation with the mother and boyfriend will be like?*
- *Will you treat them differently than other visitors?*
- *How should/would the care of the patient be different?*
- *What support systems have you identified for yourself to help you through this situation?*

As you can see, you could write this up as a case study for individuals to complete, use it for group discussion, or ask orientees to reflect on the case and write their answers to the questions.

Roles of Stakeholders (Principals)

Now that you have a better idea of what competency is and how it's measured, it's time to turn our focus onto what roles the stakeholders play in both measuring and facilitating an orientee's competency. These roles may overlap (especially as different organizations have different resources, job titles, etc.). We provide a generic description for each role, but you could easily shift these roles and responsibilities to other stakeholders.

Manager

Ultimately, the manager is the person responsible for competency assessment. Managers may delegate this responsibility to an educator or someone who observes the orientee more frequently (especially in organizations that have unit-based educators). However, from a regulatory perspective, the manager is responsible for the competency of all of his/her employees.

So, what are practical things a manager can do to assess an orientee's competency? Here are some possible activities:

- Check in with the orientee frequently and ask how she or he is feeling
- When seeing the orientee in the clinical setting, ask questions about the patient assignment to determine his/her understanding of the situation (e.g., "What's going on with your patient today?")
- Review, sign, and maintain orientation documentation upon completion of orientation
- Maintain regular communication with preceptor(s) and/or educator

It may be helpful to schedule meetings at regular intervals (for example, every 2 weeks or every month) where the manager, educator, preceptor, and orientee can also sit down together to discuss the orientee's progress. Benefits of organizing a meeting in this way include:

- Providing a more formal feedback environment

- Ensuring all primary stakeholders are on the same page
- Demonstrating to the orientee that he/she is valued enough by the manager to block out dedicated time just for that individual
- Offering an opportunity for all stakeholders to review and sign relevant orientation paperwork

Educator

In organizations with unit-based educators, those educators will likely be the primary contact persons for most orientation-related activities, including the documentation and determination of competency achievement. (For information on documentation specifics, check out Chapter 7.) Therefore, the educator will be involved in a wide variety of activities that may assist with obtaining competency but should also be used to evaluate competency. For example, an educator may teach a class for new employees, and during this time question-and-answer discussions or tests and quizzes could be used to assist with ensuring knowledge acquisition.

An educator may be involved in any of the following; however, this list is not exhaustive:

- Check in with the orientee and preceptor(s) frequently and ask how he/she is feeling
- When seeing the orientee in the clinical setting, ask questions about the patient assignment to determine his/her understanding of the situation (e.g., "What's going on with your patient today?")
- Review and sign orientation documentation from preceptor
- Aggregate all relevant documentation into one document for manager to review, sign, and file
- Maintain regular communication with preceptor(s) and manager
- Develop and deliver nonclinical learning opportunities (for example, classes, simulations, debriefing sessions)
- Assign orientee to appropriate preceptor(s)
- If time permits, act as preceptor for one or more shifts

Here are some questions that the manager and educator can use when checking with the orientee:

- *What's going on with your patient today?*
- *How's the family doing?*
- *What's keeping your patient here?*
- *What else do you have planned for the day?*
- *Are you getting the support you need to be successful with this patient?*
- *What can I do to help you?*

Preceptor

The preceptor will be the primary teacher/instructor during unit-level orientation. Because of this, the preceptor also serves as the primary evaluator of an orientee's competence. This is not an easy task; it requires skill, hard work, and compassion. Simply being an excellent clinician does not ensure you will be an excellent teacher, and many times, newer preceptors require a significant amount of professional development. Professional development specialists and managers will be essential in providing these development opportunities for preceptors.

The major responsibilities of the preceptor include:

- Collaborate with charge nurse to select patient assignments that will provide optimal learning opportunities

- Assess orientee performance on a day-to-day (or even minute-to-minute) basis

- Provide real-time feedback to orientee (both positive and constructive)

- Maintain regular communication with manager and educator

- Document relevant learning opportunities

- Review and sign final orientation document

Providing "optimal learning opportunities" can be challenging, especially in situations in which multiple orientees are on the unit at the same time or when selection of desired patients is not possible. *Mastering Precepting: A Nurse's Handbook for Success* (Ulrich, 2012) provides much greater insight and detail than we can provide here. But in an effort to provide some practical information, Worksheet 4.1 is a short worksheet that may help preceptors in choosing appropriate assignments.

WORKSHEET 4.1 *Selecting Patient Assignments to Enhance Learning Opportunities*

ORIENTEE NAME:

ASSESSMENT	CONSIDERATION FOR ASSIGNMENT
What are the orientee's primary strengths?	You probably want to avoid patient assignments that would be too easy for the orientee, because these do not provide new learning opportunities but rather reinforcement of previously acquired knowledge. (However, if an orientee is struggling with confidence, this could be appropriate to help enhance his or her self-esteem.)
What are the orientee's primary areas for improvement? (What has he/she struggled with or verbalized as being a problem?)	Selecting assignments that allow the orientee to work on areas for improvement with the assistance of his/her preceptor is ideal. Identifying these areas and transforming them into strengths are key purposes of the orientation process. Note: Sometimes you can find an assignment that allows the orientee to demonstrate his/her strength while learning or improving another competency area. This helps the orientee with confidence yet continues to develop competence.
Has the orientee recently had nonclinical learning activities such as classes or workshops?	Selecting diagnoses and procedures similar to what was covered in the nonclinical activity would help to reinforce that content and helps many orientees to have those "aha!" moments by providing the opportunity to see/touch/experience the information in real life.

ASSESSMENT	CONSIDERATION FOR ASSIGNMENT
Is there any patient with a rare diagnosis on the unit?	If less-commonly seen diagnoses or procedures are present on the unit, these could be beneficial to experience during orientation so that the first time an orientee provides care for this diagnosis or procedure is before he/she is working independently.

Documentation of relevant learning opportunities could include a wide variety of details, and Chapter 7 provides additional information. Briefly, however, a preceptor should document each shift:

- Assignment details (patient's age, diagnoses, procedures, etc.)

- Skills performed by the orientee

- Orientee's strengths and areas for improvement

Orientee

Unfortunately, it can be easy to forget the orientee's responsibility in assessing competency. The subjective experience of the orientee (as described in Table 4.1) is important in determining readiness to practice independently. Here are the activities in which the orientee should be actively participating:

- Verbalize expectations of preceptor(s), educator, and/or manager regarding what the orientee needs to feel successful

- Contribute to, review, and sign orientation documentation

- Attend and participate in all clinical and nonclinical learning opportunities

- Reflect on and share one's strengths and areas for improvement

Peers and Other Healthcare Providers

Consistent with principles of onboarding, social interactions play a huge role in the success of a new employee. Although the manager, educator, preceptor(s), and orientee may compose the group of key stakeholders, other healthcare providers (and especially their nurse peers) also play a role in successful orientation and onboarding of a new hire.

The role of others may include:

- Introducing self to orientee and getting to know him/her (even inviting him/her to social events will be helpful from an onboarding perspective)

- Providing the orientee a learning opportunity with one's patient assignment if the orientee needs that experience

- Giving feedback to preceptor(s) if the peer recognizes a strength or area for improvement

Conclusion

Assessing or evaluating competency is a huge undertaking due to its complexity; however, it is also the most pivotal moment in the orientation and onboarding process, as it will determine when an orientee can practice independently. If you use the AACN Synergy Model and Benner's competence continuum and layer your organization's definition of competence, you will have a robust understanding of what it takes to be successful.

For a nice example of one organization's approach to including many of the aforementioned models, check out Chapter 7, where we have included the worksheet that Cincinnati Children's Hospital Medical Center has developed. Their model has been designed using the theoretical underpinnings of Benner's "Novice to Expert" model, the AACN Synergy Model, and the organization's job standards and clinical ladder.

Questions for Reflection and Discussion

1. Which approach to orientation (time-based or competency-based) do you see as being optimal, and why? How could your organization transition approaches if desired?

2. Where do you see many orientees having the greatest learning curve: cognitive knowledge, psychomotor skills, affective thoughts/behaviors, interpersonal skills, or critical thinking? Is there anything you could change about your orientation program to assist with this?

3. Which stakeholders in your organization have the largest involvement in an orientee's training and evaluation? Should those who have the least involvement become more involved, and is there anything they could learn from those who have the largest involvement?

KEY TAKEAWAYS

- *Competency-based orientation programs ensure that orientees are competent and haven't just spent the right amount of time in orientation and onboarding.*
- *Evaluating competency is a multi-faceted process.*
- *Competency assessment should consider cognitive knowledge, psychomotor skills, and affective thoughts and behaviors.*
- *Ensure key stakeholders play active roles in evaluating competency.*

References

Benner, P. (1982). From novice to expert. *The American Journal of Nursing, 82*(3), 402-407.

Benner, P. (2004). Using the Dreyfus model of skill acquisition to describe and interpret skill acquisition and clinical judgment in nursing practice and education. *Bulletin of Science, Technology, & Society, 24*(3), 188-199.

Goleman, D. (2006). *Emotional Intelligence: Why it can matter more than IQ* (10th Anniversary ed.). New York, NY: Bantam.

Insight Assessment. (2013). *Health sciences reasoning test.* Retrieved from http://www.insightassessment.com

Ulrich, B. (2012). *Mastering precepting: A nurse's handbook for success.* Indianapolis, IN: Sigma Theta Tau International.

CHAPTER 5

Working With Orientees

Introduction

Orientees will come to you with a wide variety of experiences, both personally and professionally, and the approach you take to working with them may vary just as much. Although the outcome of orientation should be the same for all nurses on the unit (providing safe and competent care), how the orientee travels through orientation may be unique. This chapter will focus on how to manage a variety of common orientee scenarios and help you develop strategies for working with them.

If you're short on time, you're welcome to jump to the page that discusses your particular situation. Are you working with an orientee who:

- Is a new graduate nurse? (p. 98)

- Is an experienced nurse? (p. 101)

- Is progressing quickly? (p. 102)

- Made an error? (p. 104)

- Has a personality conflict with his/her preceptor? (p. 107)

- Has a learning style that doesn't match his/her preceptor's teaching style? (p. 109)

- Struggles with interpersonal communication? (p. 110)

- Wants to quit? (p. 112)

- Can't successfully complete orientation? (p. 114)

The New Graduate Nurse

New graduate (NG) nurses are, by far, the most predictable in their journeys. Even though their clinical and academic preparation may vary, they do not enter the professional realm with their own independent nursing experience upon which they can make decisions. They are like moldable clay that can be transformed into whatever you and your unit desire. Hopefully, that is both exciting and a little bit scary to you!

REAL-WORLD EXAMPLE: MOLDABLE MOLLY

Molly just started as an NG nurse on the unit. She is excited about being a nurse, but she is quite nervous about coming into work every day. Molly's preceptors have no concerns with her performance.

Molly goes to her educator and manager frequently with reports of, "I feel like I'm not getting it. I'm too slow, and I think I'm missing things. Everything seems so easy to my preceptor, and I've noticed that my friends are getting done with tasks faster than I am."

Molly is the typical NG nurse. She has enthusiasm and excitement while meeting the expectations of her preceptors. However, her confidence level is low. Nurses whose competence is on target but whose confidence is low require encouragement, support, listening, and guided reflection. Provide frequent positive comments and focus on their strengths and the areas in which they have demonstrated great improvement. Listen to their concerns and let them know confidence is one of the last feelings NG nurses acquire. Providing opportunities for reflection (both through in-person dialogue and journaling) will help them move more efficiently toward healthy self-confidence.

Encourage them not to compare themselves to their peers. They probably don't see how much their peers are actually doing, and

The Experienced Nurse

Experienced nurses are those nurses who have had at least 9 to 12 months of providing patient care outside of their academic training. Experience can span a wide variety of years as well as specialties, and although an experienced nurse has established the foundations of critical thinking (and hopefully psychomotor skill), moving to a new specialty can be overwhelming. The greater the change in specialty, the more difficult the transition may be (e.g., transitioning from adult hospice to pediatric critical care will be a larger change than transitioning from a medical intensive care unit to a surgical intensive care unit).

REAL-WORLD EXAMPLE: EXPERIENCED ELEANORE

Eleanore has 5 years of experience working with telemetry patients in an adult hospital. She has decided that she would like to work with children, so she has taken a job in a neonatal intensive care unit.

Eleanore's preceptors note that she is slow to document and respond to patient alarms, but there are no issues with medication administration or patient assessments. Eleanore tells her educator and manager, "The babies are just so much smaller than I'm used to. I have no problem giving out the medications, but my preceptor keeps telling me I'm not prioritizing correctly."

Your role in staff development will be to help the orientee (and the preceptor) identify knowledge gaps and learning opportunities to bridge those gaps. Whether those opportunities are classes, self-directed reading and studying, or patient assignments, selecting the best learning activities for an experienced nurse will be key in his/her success. Chances are high that if the experienced nurse was successful in a previous organization or department, he/she will be successful in yours, given the appropriate guidance and learning opportunities.

If you are working with preceptors who are more familiar with NG nurses, the preceptors may need to be reminded that experienced nurses develop differently than NG nurses because they have experiences that have shaped their approach to patient care and decision-making. If decision-making (regarding things such as time management and prioritization) needs to occur differently than it did in their previous environment, the preceptor will need to identify these differences and attempt to verbalize what may be unspoken or implicit knowledge among nurses in the department. For example, the preceptors should verbally state, "If you're short on time, the medical team would like to see vital signs and physical assessment charted before intake and output," or "Don't put your whole lunch box in the refrigerator because if everyone does that on day shift, it takes up too much space. Try to place only cold items in there."

Consult Table 5.2 for some of the behaviors you might see from an experienced nurse orientee and appropriate actions you can take.

TABLE 5.2 *Behaviors and Response for Experienced Nurse Orientees*

BEHAVIORS	RESPONSE
Experienced Eleanore	**Guiding Gail**
Basic nursing skills mastered & specialty nursing skills quickly acquired	Assist orientee in integrating these basic & specialty skills
Uses previous experiences/methods for managing time & priorities	Verbalize implicit/unspoken behaviors & group thought processes

The Quickly Progressing Nurse

Some nurses will progress through orientation more quickly than the average new hire. For NG nurses this can be a result of receiving greater academic and/or clinical preparation, entering the workplace with more life experience, or having an increased capacity for cognitive and/or emotional intelligence. For experienced nurses, a quicker progression will more likely occur if their previous environment is similar to the new one.

REAL-WORLD EXAMPLE: QUICK QUINTON

Quinton is a new graduate orientee in an outpatient orthopedic clinic who is well liked and respected by current staff, including the surgeons and management. Quinton tells his educator, "I'm feeling good about things, and I really like it here."

Allie is also a new graduate who started with Quinton, and she is right on track with completing orientation in the expected time allotment. There are no issues with her performance, but she tends to be shy in social settings and doesn't personally know the staff as well as Quinton does. Allie repeatedly says to her preceptor, "I'm just not getting it. It's all too much for me, and I don't feel like I'm doing anything right. Maybe this place isn't for me."

Once the quickly progressing orientee builds a reputation for "catching on quickly," the preceptors and peers may assume he/she knows more than he/she actually does. Although it is important to acknowledge progression and competency, learning is a never-ending process in healthcare, and there is always additional information that the new hire could benefit from learning. Staff development specialists should remind preceptors not to decrease their rigor while evaluating continued progress. Preceptors may need additional training in how to verbally structure their teaching moments in such a way that acknowledges the new hire's proficiency while simultaneously offering potentially new or forgotten information. For example, instead of asking, "Have you done [insert skill] before?" it may be better to ask, "What has been your experience with [insert skill]?" This allows for a wider variety of responses rather than simply a "yes/no."

If several new hires start orientation at the same time (such as a cohort), some may begin to feel their performance is inadequate compared to the quickly progressing orientee. This is most notable with NG cohorts and needs to be handled delicately. Requiring significantly more positive reinforcement than their experienced counterparts, NG nurses frequently compare themselves with the peers in their cohort to self-assess their progress. When they see other orientees progressing more quickly or finishing orientation earlier, the average or slower-progressing orientee may have profound episodes of self-doubt and begin to frequently ask what is wrong with their practice.

Tables 5.3 and 5.4 cover some behaviors and appropriate responses when you are dealing both with quickly progressing orientees and their peers, who might be progressing at a slower, albeit normal, pace.

TABLE 5.3 *Behaviors and Response for Quickly Progressing Orientees*

BEHAVIORS	RESPONSE
Quick Quinton	**Consistent Connie**
Reaches milestones ahead of time	Recognize accomplishments
Well-liked by other staff	Encourage continued socialization/onboarding
Labeled as an "easy orientee" by preceptor	Maintain consistent, rigorous evaluation standards equivalent to those of other orientees
	Ask open-ended questions that acknowledge expertise while also creating a potential learning opportunity

TABLE 5.4 *Behaviors and Response for the Peers of Quickly Progressing Orientees*

BEHAVIORS	RESPONSE
Average Allie	**Refocusing Riley**
No performance issues	Reaffirm strengths
Frequently questions self-progress	Focus on growth
Mentions peers' action more than own	Redirect attention to orientee's performance

When Orientees Make Errors

All healthcare providers, regardless of profession, specialty, and experience level, are at risk for making errors. Just as the title of the Institute of Medicine (2000) report so appropriately stated, *To Err is Human*. Making an error may become even easier when a clinician is exposed to a new environment that requires a new set of competencies. Therefore, errors are not uncommon during the orientation period, and you need to balance the normalcy of making errors with the excellent learning opportunity they present.

REAL-WORLD EXAMPLE: MED MIX-UP MELANIE

Melanie is a new nurse in a long-term care facility in which the rooms are designed such that two patients can be present in the same room. Melanie was administering medications one morning before breakfast to two patients who required different doses of insulin, and she administered the wrong dose to both of them.

The patient who received too much insulin collapsed to the floor when getting up to use the restroom. The patient quickly regained consciousness and was placed back in bed, where her glucose was normalized with oral, sugar-containing fluids. She had no long-term injuries.

Errors can occur in a wide variety of situations, and their impact severity can range from near-miss to death. The approach to working with an orientee who has made an error will be largely influenced by the scope and impact of the error.

In Melanie's case, the error resulted in temporary harm to the patient. If Melanie were a new graduate (or experienced but with little confidence at this point), this error could be devastating to her self-confidence. Therefore, the preceptor (as well as other supporting players such as the staff development specialist, manager, peers, etc.) needs to assess the orientee's feelings of the situation. You can start by using Gibbs's reflective cycle (see Figure 5.1) and accompanying questions (Gibbs, 1988). Depending on the orientee's reaction to the situation, the supporting persons may need to help Melanie focus on the involvement of various systems factors (such as room design, the medication administration process, etc.) in the error occurrence. This can help Melanie understand how one can be prone to errors.

If the error would have resulted in more severe harm to the patient, professional counseling may be required, and the organization should provide assistance in receiving this support. Conversely, if the error did not reach the patient (a near-miss), the preceptor should seek to determine if the orientee understands the impact this "close call" could have had.

Regardless of the impact on confidence, the error should always be used as a learning opportunity. Many newer nurses will cope with the situation by developing a mentality that will make them hyperaware of the precipitating factors in the future. Some paraphrase this mind-set by stating, "Well, I know I will never do that again!"

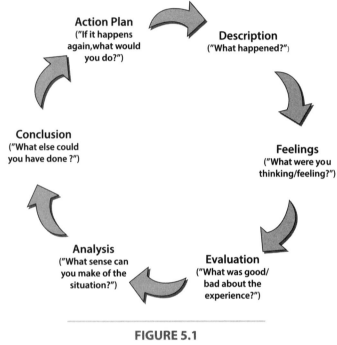

FIGURE 5.1

Gibbs's Reflective Cycle.

Finally, all errors, including near-misses, should be communicated to the appropriate risk management personnel in the organization, who can look into preventing this from happening in the future.

Table 5.5 suggests appropriate responses to keep in mind when orientees make errors.

TABLE 5.5 *Behaviors and Response for Orientees Who Make an Error*

BEHAVIORS	RESPONSE
Med Mix-Up Melanie	**Comforting & Clarifying Cathy**
Preoccupied with the error	Care for patient immediately after event
Decreased confidence	Comfort orientee
Concerned about making the same mistake again	Discuss strategies for doing it correctly

Personality Conflicts

Regardless of the skill and expertise of the assigned preceptor, personality conflicts are bound to arise during the orientation period. Orientees and preceptors can vary in their experience level, educational background, gender, race, culture, values, and social norms. Although nurses may possess great skill in taking care of patients who differ from them, it can become quite stressful for a preceptor to both care for patients while also working with a new hire. This may be comparable to taking on two sets of patients concurrently. Additionally, the orientees are under a high degree of stress simply by the massive learning trajectory they face.

When these stressors are placed in the context of a complex healthcare environment, it may be difficult to adapt and "keep your cool" when faced with what appears to be an impossible task. The capacity to be empathetic and patient is diminished in these situations, and incompatible personalities in the teacher-learner dyad further complicate the problem.

REAL-WORLD EXAMPLE: PERSONALITY PROBLEM PAULA

Paula is a new graduate nurse in a psychiatric hospital whose preceptor, Alan, is very concerned that "she just isn't getting it." The staff development specialist has met with Paula and feels that she isn't progressing as quickly as she should be but is fairly confident she has the knowledge and skills needed to be successful.

Alan has been caught raising his voice at Paula and even slapping her hand as Paula is about to perform a small task incorrectly. Both Paula and Alan get very frustrated when their patient assignment is busy or when high acuity situations occur. Paula states, "Alan is just so mean and doesn't teach me anything beneficial. I don't think he likes me."

Ideally, preceptors and orientees should be paired by complementary personality styles, if known. This could be achieved by soliciting input from someone who personally knows both of them, or by using select personality tools (for example, the Myers-Briggs Type Indicator [MBTI] or Keirsey Temperament Sorter).

If it is not possible to match them (either due to not knowing the orientee or not having a large enough preceptor pool) or if this matching was not successful, additional assessments should be performed to uncover the cause of the conflicting personalities. The preceptor and orientee need to verbalize their natural tendencies regarding communication and decision-making so that the conversation becomes open to discuss these differences. This is one of those "easier said than done" activities that may benefit from having a mediator present, such as a staff development specialist.

The staff development specialist should bring the preceptor and the orientee together in a quiet meeting space. The purpose of the meeting is to help create a proper line of communication. Questions to use for the meeting include:

- How do you like to give feedback? Receive feedback?
- How do you like to receive praise? Constructive criticism?
- What is your favorite thing about your job?
- What is your least favorite thing about your job?
- What are your pet peeves and/or hot buttons?
- What ground rules would you propose to keep the lines of communication open with this other person?

The staff development specialist can give them some silent time for each to make notes about his/her response to the questions, and then the specialist would facilitate a discussion about their answers and get them to agree to ground rules moving forward.

If none of these interventions resolve the problem, it may be necessary to assign the orientee to a different preceptor. Managers and educators should reinforce to the preceptor that irreconcilable differences do occur, and successful orientation of the new hire is the priority. However, this may also be an opportunity for professional development of the preceptor, and after assessing his/her behaviors and communication styles, he/she may learn new approaches for working with orientees in the future.

Alvin's experience has been that preceptors initially may be upset by the decision to place their orientees with someone else. However, those preceptors are frequently thankful for that decision by the end of the new hires' orientation period once they see the various challenges the new preceptor-orientee pairs faced.

Table 5.6 can help you spot the behaviors and respond appropriately when preceptors and orientees have personality conflicts.

TABLE 5.6 *Behaviors and Response for Orientees Who Have a Personality Conflict With Preceptor*

BEHAVIORS	RESPONSE
Personality Problem Paula	**Adaptable Alan**
Easily frustrated	Display patience
Not receptive to feedback	Investigate orientee's preferred method for learning and receiving feedback
Speaks poorly of preceptor to others	Verbalize desire for orientee's success

Teaching/Learning Style Conflicts

Many of the concepts found in working with personality conflicts also hold true with teaching/learning style conflict. In fact, it can be difficult, initially, to determine if the frustrations of a preceptor and/or orientee are due to a true personality conflict or, more simply, if the orientee has a learning style the preceptor is not considering when teaching.

As in personality conflict, the most ideal situation is to match preceptors and orientees with similar learning styles. If the preceptor has a similar learning style, he/she is more likely to teach in a way that is easily received by the orientee. Several available tools can assess learning styles, including but not limited to: Kolb, MBTI, and VARK (see Chapter 2 for more information).

If pairing similar learning styles is not possible, preceptor development and training can prove very beneficial. By assisting the preceptor in modifying his/her preferred teaching style based on the orientee's learning style, orientees will acquire the necessary knowledge and skills in a shorter period of time and (hopefully) with less frustration on the part of the preceptor.

For preceptors who have not had formal training in education strategies, it can be easy to assume that all people learn in a similar manner as they do. Alvin has frequently heard nurses say, "We learn by being hands-on, not by reading it or hearing about it." Although the majority of nurses may be sensory, and even more specifically, kinesthetic learners (Frankel, 2009; Smith, 2010), not all nurses can be placed into this category, and effective preceptors will adapt their teaching styles to their orientees' learning styles.

Struggling With Interpersonal Communication

Although nurses receive training on skillful and therapeutic communication during their academic preparation, activities such as active listening and carefully selecting the right words to say may be more difficult to apply when communicating with a coworker rather than a patient. The peer-peer and preceptor-orientee relationships can be quite different from the nurse-patient relationship. Workplace relationships are longer lasting, and the capacity for patience and empathy may not be as great toward their peers. This can be complicated by unit/department culture and social norms, many of which will be new to an orientee.

REAL-WORLD EXAMPLE: DEFENSIVE DAN

Dan is an experienced nurse who recently transferred to the trauma-surgical intensive care unit from a medical intensive care unit in a nearby hospital. When his preceptor attempts to provide feedback about his performance, Dan regularly responds harshly, and he has been known to simply walk away.

Dan tells his educator, "I don't think people like me here. It's like people don't want me to do well here, and they always are criticizing me." As the educator performs follow-up, discussions with the preceptor, Gina, reveal that it can be very challenging for Gina to give Dan feedback about his performance and that Dan is resistant to being taught skills that are performed differently from his previous institution.

Many of the concepts discussed in the personality conflict section apply to this situation, too. In fact, it can be difficult to differentiate between personality conflicts and communication struggles as a person's communication style can be influenced by his/her temperament and character. The most important component of managing interpersonal communication challenges in the preceptor-orientee relationship will be to discuss openly the expectations of both parties. This may involve answering questions like:

- When does the orientee prefer to receive feedback (for example, in real time or at the end of the shift)?

- Where should feedback be provided (for example, in the patient's room, at the nurse's station, or in a break room)?

- How will expectations for the day (or week) be established and evaluated?

- How much involvement does the orientee expect of the preceptor?

While this conversation can be mediated by a third party if requested, honestly discussing expectations and mutually agreeing upon acceptable behaviors will be fundamental to creating an environment in which the orientee has the optimal learning opportunity.

Most interpersonal communication struggles will occur between healthcare providers; however, some new hires may struggle in communicating with patients and families. Hopefully, this was identified and addressed during the academic program. However, the stresses of a new work environment may make it difficult for a new hire to communicate appropriately with patients and families. If this is the case, the orientee should first be told that patients and families perceive his/her communication as inappropriate or difficult to understand. Many times, simply stating this perception will be enough for the new hire to admit to an elevated stress level, which then opens the discussion for establishing healthy coping mechanisms and, eventually, effective communication strategies.

For an orientee who does not see a need to change his/her communication style, the manager should be brought quickly into the discussion to determine if the employee's skill set and professional goals are a good match for the organization's mission and vision. If an incongruence surfaces, you may want to jump to the section "Unable to Successfully Complete Orientation" later in the chapter.

Table 5.7 shows the signs of an orientee having communication struggles and suggests what you can do about it.

TABLE 5.7 *Behaviors and Response for Orientees Who Struggle with Interpersonal Communication*

BEHAVIORS	RESPONSE
Defensive Dan	**Gentle Gina**
May not be receptive to feedback	Investigate orientee's preferred method for learning and receiving feedback
Quick or "hot" tempered at times	
Verbalizes feelings of "not fitting in"	Display patience
Doesn't engage in socialization opportunities	Facilitate socialization by engaging both orientee and peers

Wanting to Quit

Some literature suggests the percentage of new graduate nurses who choose to leave their first job within their first year is as great as 60% (Godinez, Schweiger, Gruver, & Ryan, 1999). Ideally, implementing recommendations from this book and other sources will help you and your organization keep your first-year turnover rate far below this mark. However, even under ideal situations with optimal work environments and healthy interpersonal relationships, some new hires may simply not enjoy the specific patient population for whom your department provides nursing care.

> **REAL-WORLD EXAMPLE: DISINTERESTED DEREK**
>
> *Derek started working in the surgical intensive care unit of a large urban medical center as a new graduate nurse. He previously worked in the unit as an administrative assistant during nursing school, and he had many clinical experiences in the neighboring medical intensive care unit. During nursing school, he frequently questioned whether or not he wanted to work in the unit as a nurse. He executed his administrative assistant duties with superb ratings, and his coworkers convinced him that he should pursue a nursing position after graduation.*
>
> *During orientation, Derek acquired his skills quickly and got along well with his preceptor. However, he struggled a bit with confidence and continued to question whether or not this was the right place for him. Toward the end of orientation, after being exposed to a wide variety of patient experiences, he verbalized to his manager, "I just don't think this place is for me. I didn't realize how sick these patients can get, and I don't think I like my patients being this ill."*

Begin your assessment of the situation with ensuring that the orientee truly dislikes the patient population as opposed to some other aspect of the work environment, or conflicts or issues such as those mentioned in previous sections of this chapter. Pending no other identified problems, working with an orientee who simply does not find fulfillment (or outright hates) caring for the patient population in your area can be a challenge.

Ideally, the hiring process ensures candidates who are not truly passionate about the selected patient population are not hired. However, even the best talent acquisition processes may allow some candidates through the cracks. This is especially true of new graduate orientees who may not know themselves what their desired patient population is yet.

Once this desire to leave is confirmed, guidance from Human Resources may be needed to assist with the next steps. Some organizations do not allow new hires to transfer to another department within their probationary period. Because it is likely that the probationary period cannot be completed until orientation is wrapped up, the orientee may have to successfully complete orientation and begin caring for patients in your department until their probationary period is done.

Additionally, transferring within the organization early in one's career may look suspicious to the department to which the new hire is applying to work. The staff development specialist and/or manager can assist with this transition by writing a letter of recommendation, commenting on the orientee's proficiency in caring for the patient population, and explaining the situation, if the orientee requests such a letter. (Please check with Human Resources before writing recommendation letters for other employees to ensure compliance with organizational guidelines.)

Finally, preceptors should be reassured that the orientee's desire to leave is in no way a reflection of the preceptor's performance but rather a personal choice to work with a different patient population.

Consult Table 5.8 to prepare yourself for behaviors you might see from orientees who want to quit and to ready yourself to respond.

TABLE 5.8 *Behaviors and Response for Orientees Who Want to Quit*

BEHAVIORS	RESPONSE
Disinterested Derek	**Understanding Ursula**
No performance issues	Reaffirm strengths
High stress level and/or low confidence	Emphasize orientee's positive impact on patient/family
Verbalizes desire to quit	Listen and assist with decision-making

Orientees Unable to Successfully Complete Orientation

Probably the most challenging and least desirable of all orientation situations is when a new hire is unable to successfully complete orientation. Even though all nurses complete comparable academic studies and pass the same national licensure exam, not every individual's combination of knowledge, skills, attitudes, and decision-making styles is appropriate for the patient population and/or organization with whom he/she chooses to work.

REAL-WORLD EXAMPLE: STRUGGLING STACI

Staci is a new graduate nurse in the operating room whom all the staff adore. She is kind to all patients and peers, and she communicates effectively. However, multiple safety incidents have resulted from her performance, including many near-misses and even a couple of events that resulted in temporary harm to the patient. All of these events were reviewed with her, and additional training was provided. Yet, some behaviors resulted in repeated events.

Staci tells her educator, "I promise I'm trying because I really do want to work here. I just don't understand how all of this keeps happening." Staci is tearful during these conversations.

For the nurses serving as the preceptors, managers, and staff development specialists, one of the most difficult challenges is listening to more than the caring and compassionate voice inside you that says,

"But she's really sweet. She might eventually get it." As nurses, we possess a great ability for seeing and appreciating the value of every human being. Although this skill is necessary in caring for people whom we identify as patients, it can make it difficult for us to objectively evaluate people whom we identify as peers or colleagues.

Early signs of inadequate performance may be noticed at the beginning of orientation, but it will likely take some time to determine that an employee may need to be terminated. No new hire enters the organization without the need for at least some training and orientation, but some employees will reach a point at which additional training will not provide sufficient assistance for them to work independently in a safe and effective manner.

Identifying the point at which training will no longer be beneficial is complicated. Some organizations have a standard length of orientation, and orientees who cannot complete orientation within that designated time are terminated. Other organizations have a competency-based approach, and the educator and manager may have to rely on the average of previous new hires' orientation times to decide when the process is taking too long.

When you are concerned that an orientee may not be able to successfully complete orientation, you should try to determine the factors preventing him/her from being successful (which are hopefully discussed earlier in this chapter) and alleviate those problems. Manager involvement should be solicited at the moment you are concerned because if all efforts to improve performance prove unsuccessful, it will be the manager's responsibility to coordinate the termination process. More information about the legal aspects of terminating a new hire can be found in Chapter 7 of this book.

Regardless of the process and speed of termination, the preceptor should continue to focus on incorporating strategies mentioned elsewhere in this text in an attempt to correct or improve performance issues. These continued efforts to provide a successful orientation experience may eventually give the orientee what he/she needs to "turn the corner" and maintain employment. In all circumstances, however, detailed documentation of preceptor efforts and orientee responses is essential.

Table 5.9 goes over the behaviors of orientees who can't successfully complete orientation and your possible responses to that situation.

TABLE 5.9 *Behaviors and Response for Orientees Who Are Unable to Successfully Complete Orientation*

BEHAVIORS	RESPONSE
Struggling Staci	**Persistent Patrick**
Significant performance issues but potentially unaware of them	Continue teaching and providing feedback
Will likely verbalize desire to improve and may go "above and beyond" with some tasks to demonstrate competency	Acknowledge orientee's efforts Document preceptor interventions and orientee behaviors in detail
May be easily frustrated with tasks	Maintain frequent communication with manager and/or educator

Conclusion

Orientees come in a wide variety of shapes and sizes, and the interventions required to transform them into safe and effective clinicians can be just as varied. Especially for those orientees who do not follow a "typical" pathway through orientation, identifying their challenges may not be as simple as represented in this chapter. Additionally, some orientees may fit in somewhere between these classifications and require pick-and-choose interventions from different categories. Whatever struggles arise, open communication and strong collaboration between all involved parties will be essential to the orientee's success.

Questions for Reflection/Discussion

1. What academic preparation do your typical new graduate nursing orientees have?

2. How prepared is your orientation program for new graduate nurses who do not have the typical academic preparation the rest of your orientees have?

3. Which of the listed orientee types is most prevalent in your unit, department, or organization?

4. Which of the listed orientee types would be easiest and which most difficult for you (the professional development specialist) to manage? Why?

5. Which of the listed orientee types is most difficult for your staff members (direct care providers, preceptors, charge nurses, etc.) to work with? Why?

6. What preparation do your preceptors have to manage these various orientee types?

7. What preparation do your managers have to manage these various orientee types?

KEY TAKEAWAYS

- *Orientees come with a wide array of backgrounds, personalities, and characteristics, and your approach to working with them will vary just as much.*
- *There is not a "one size fits all" approach to any specific orientee consideration, but you will begin to see themes and patterns after you work with them long enough. Until then, try some of the approaches we have outlined in this chapter.*
- *Creating an orientation program that has an ample amount of flexibility will be beneficial in successfully accommodating a variety of orientees.*
- *Open lines of communication among the staff development specialist, the orientee, the preceptor, and the hiring manager are critical to the success of any onboarding process.*

References

Frankel, A. (2009). Nurses' learning styles: Promoting better integration of theory into practice. *Nursing Times, 105*(2), 24-27.

Gibbs, G. (1988). Learning by doing: A guide to teaching and learning methods. Oxford, England: Oxford Polytechnic.

Godinez, G., Schweiger, J., Gruver, J., & Ryan, P. (1999). Role transition from graduate to staff nurse: A qualitative analysis. *Journal for Nurses in Staff Development, 15*(3), 97-110.

Institute of Medicine (IOM). (2000). *To err is human: Building a safer health system.* Washington, DC: National Academy Press.

Krugman, M., Bretschneider, J., Horn, P. B., Krsek, C. A., Moutafis, R. A., & Smith, M. O. (2006). The national post-baccalaureate graduate nurse residency program: A model for excellence in transition to practice. *Journal for Nurses in Staff Development, 22*(4), 196-205.

Pine, R., & Tart, K. (2007). Return on investment: Benefits and challenges of a baccalaureate nurse residency program. *Nursing Economic$, 25*(1), 13-18, 39.

Smith, A. (2010). Learning styles of registered nurses enrolled in an online nursing program. *Journal of Professional Nursing, 26*(1), 49-53. doi: 10.1016/j.profnurs.2009.04.006

CHAPTER 6

Evaluating an Orientation Program

Introduction

Orientation programs, regardless of their design or structure, should be evaluated for their efficacy. Just as the nursing process and ADDIE model complete their cycles with *Evaluation*, so do all successful programs. By evaluating your orientation program from various perspectives and levels, you ensure an effective, efficient orientation program that adds value to the individual, the unit/department, and the organization...a win-win-win situation.

Evaluating an orientation program should provide you with useful information that will do one of two things:

1. Describe areas of the program that need to be modified because they are not as effective or efficient as they could be, or

2. Supply evidence that the program is, in fact, doing what it's supposed to do

Although this may sound simple and self-evident, consider the following two examples in which having documented, objective evaluation data proved useful.

REAL-WORLD EXAMPLE: THE NEED FOR EVALUATION #1

Dan was the staff development specialist in charge of the first week of nursing orientation for all new hires entering his organization. When he assumed this role, he discovered that evaluation of this first week of training was performed by a simple survey on the last day of the week that asked these new hires if they liked the content they learned. Although Dan knew this was a good start, he felt more should be done to evaluate his program. So, he developed a survey for preceptors to complete within the first 2 weeks a new hire spent on the unit taking care of patients. This survey evaluated basic skills observed by the preceptor.

Dan quickly discovered that documentation in the electronic medical record was a problem among new hires in most departments. Therefore, he modified the training day on documentation to include more case-based and simulation scenarios. Postintervention data revealed improved documentation performance, and anecdotal feedback came to him from unit-based educators who said the new hires' ability to document efficiently had drastically increased preceptor satisfaction and allowed them to cover more advanced skills much earlier.

This example shows how including various levels of evaluation provides for a more well-rounded assessment of program efficacy and highlights potential opportunities for improvement.

REAL-WORLD EXAMPLE: THE NEED FOR EVALUATION #2

Marie, a unit-based educator, was invited to attend a meeting with other unit-based educators as well as several senior-level managers who had a strong influence on training and development in the organization. Due to economic hardships, the managers informed the educators that various "nonessential" components of initial orientation would be removed. Notably, an 8-hour class on medication safety was being removed from central orientation based on the rationale that licensed healthcare providers should already be familiar with this information, and preceptors should be reinforcing it at the unit level.

Although Marie had a "gut feeling" that this class should not be removed (and she knew that her own new hires found this class beneficial), she knew she would need more objective data to prevent the removal of the class. After the meeting, Marie gathered already-available data on rates of serious adverse drug events starting with data collected approximately 2 years before the medication safety class was added to central orientation. Marie shared the data with managers and showed them how implementation of this class resulted in a 50% decrease of serious adverse drug events and saved the organization more money than what was spent on salary for attending the class. The managers decided to keep this class in orientation.

This example shows the value of collecting objective evaluation data for the purpose of maintaining orientation components that have proven value.

Alvin's experience in teaching project management strategies to nurses has revealed that objectively evaluating a project or program does not come naturally for many nurses. Evaluation of a program (or even a change in a program) should stem from the assessment data that warranted its presence. Unfortunately, many nurses settle for a level of evaluation as simple as satisfaction with the program, even though the program was created due to a problem noted with patient care. These various levels of evaluation will be discussed throughout the chapter, but first we want to provide you with an example that will hopefully hit home.

We want to share this example as a way of showing the parallels between evaluating an orientation program and a patient's pain.

EVALUATING A PROGRAM IS LIKE EVALUATING A PATIENT'S PAIN

Consider the case of a 35-year-old patient with multiple rib fractures due to a motor vehicle accident. The patient is in pain because of the presence of a chest tube as well as movement of his ribs while breathing. He rates his pain as an 8 out of 10 on the numeric rating scale, and you (as the nurse) provide him with a standard adult dose of intravenous morphine. Which of the following sets of questions would be most valuable for evaluating the effectiveness of the pain medication after administration?

QUESTION SET A	QUESTION SET B
On a scale of 0-10, how satisfied are you with my ability to administer a pain medication?	On a scale of 0-10, how would you rate your pain now?
Do you think your pain level has changed as a result of the administering of this medication?	Is the pain level you're experiencing now manageable?
Would you recommend this pain medication to other patients?	Do you need additional help in managing your pain?

Obviously, Question Set B is the appropriate response.

Nurses are phenomenal at assessing and reassessing pain, and they are focused on one major goal—keeping the patient as comfortable as possible. As the patient's pain increases, an intervention is carried out, and the nurse reassesses to ensure the pain has decreased. Similarly, if there is a performance issue in the organization, and a new component were added in orientation to address this performance issue, the best evaluation would involve assessing the continued presence of the performance issue (not whether new hires enjoyed the training or scored better on a test).

We're not trying to minimize the importance of evaluating satisfaction with an orientation program; however, we want you to realize that evaluating an orientation program should not stop at this first level. Appropriate evaluation will relate back to the assessment data that initially suggested the need for the intervention's creation. We hope you'll keep this in mind as you read this chapter.

Levels and Types of Evaluation

Several models are used in business and education for evaluating the efficacy of a program or project, but Kirkpatrick's Four Levels of Evaluation is probably the most notable and the one from which many other evaluation models originate.

Kirkpatrick's Four Levels of Evaluation

The reason for widespread use of Kirkpatrick's model is primarily due to the simplicity and practicality of his approach (Kirkpatrick, 1996). His four levels are: reaction, learning, behavior, and results. Pros and cons of each level are listed in Table 6.1, and you can see examples of how to apply each of these levels to actual programs in Table 6.2.

Reaction

The first level, reaction, deals with the learner's reaction to the training program (what his/her experience was like during the activity). Assessment of this level could include any aspect of the program from speaker, to content and environment, to delivery style. This level of evaluation provides insight into learner satisfaction. Many training and development professionals refer to this level of evaluation as "smiley sheets." As many of you are probably aware, if content isn't delivered in a way that makes it interesting to the learner, there is little chance that the learner will put forth any effort to absorb the information (Kirkpatrick, 1996).

The reaction level of evaluation is commonly acquired in training programs due to its ease of measurement and the ability to make quick changes based on feedback. It should be delivered relatively soon after a program is delivered because participants may quickly forget things like how conducive the room was to learning.

Learning

The next level, learning, assesses how well knowledge is transferred to the learner. This could include learning in any of the cognitive, psychomotor, and even affective (attitude) domains (Kirkpatrick, 1996). While the first level asks participants for their perspective of the program, learning will be a more objective assessment that is typically measured through written tests and/or observation.

This level of evaluation is slightly more complex than the reaction level of evaluation, but it is still fairly simple to design and quite common in training programs. For example, anyone who has participated in a continuing education program online and taken a test at the end regarding the content has had their learning assessed. The best way to measure learning would be to provide pre- and post-program tests and calculate the difference between the two scores. Also, it is possible to assess learning through simulations and/or case studies.

Behavior

At this third level, evaluation begins to become much more difficult. Evaluating the level of behavior involves what Kirkpatrick (1996) refers to as transfer of training. To assess this level of evaluation, you must observe behavioral changes in the learner in his or her actual job setting. A challenge with this level is that you do not have control of what the learner encounters in the real-world setting.

For example, if you delivered a program on pressure ulcer reduction, you might want to observe whether or not nurses are turning patients at the appropriate frequency as well as their use of pressure-relieving equipment. If they are not, then you might want to see what is preventing them from following what they know to be the correct procedure and frequency. Are there environmental factors that prohibit them from doing it at the right frequency? Are there issues with the equipment they are using? Or are they simply not following the procedure they learned in the program?

NOTE ═══════════════════════════════════════

Robin had an interesting experience rolling out a project management training program at a previous employer. People were given pre- and post-tests and showed a great deal of skill improvement. Robin wanted to see how they were applying those skills on the job and conducted a qualitative (anecdotal) survey. She asked one project manager how his leader liked the weekly reports recommended in the training program. He responded, "The first time I sent a report to my manager, he told me that he never wanted to see one of them again. So, I stopped sending them." We hope that this is not happening in clinical settings, but the example does allow you to see how environment and leaders can wreak havoc on great training you have delivered!

═══

Results

The final level, results, may be the only level in which senior-level leaders are interested. Although this is definitely important, Kirkpatrick (1996) warns against *only* evaluating this level, stating that as many levels as possible should be evaluated because each provides a different perspective into a training program. When evaluating results, you are looking for the final products of a training program. These could include, but are not limited to:

- Improved quality of care

- Reduction in costs

- Increased job satisfaction (and more importantly, reduced staff turnover)

- Any metrics/indicators the organization reports to external agencies (for example, pressure ulcers or fall rates)

TABLE 6.1 *Comparison of Kirkpatrick's Four Levels of Evaluation*

	PROS	CONS
Reaction	Easy to measure Easy to make quick changes Assists in determining learner satisfaction and motivation	Does not provide an objective assessment of knowledge transfer
Learning	Relatively simple to create the instrument Quick and easy to gather data Provides an objective assessment of knowledge transfer	Does not ensure knowledge is transferred to on-the-job behaviors
Behavior	Higher level of evaluation that assesses application/use of training concepts Potentially serves as an opportunity for the observer to correct behaviors in real time	Resource-consuming (time spent observing behavior) Does not ensure the program will have an impact on desired outcome (e.g., patient care or cost savings)
Results	Likely to be of greatest interest to senior-level leaders who manage the budget and other resources	Complex Resource-consuming (both time and money)

TABLE 6.2 *Examples of Using Kirkpatrick's Four Levels of Evaluation*

Scenario: Imagine you are given the task of assessing the effectiveness of an entire orientation program for new graduate nurses in an adult medical-surgical unit. The following questions are possible measurements that could be used to assess the various levels of evaluation.

Reaction	According to a Likert scale (for example, on a scale of 1-5 [from Strongly Disagree to Strongly Agree]) survey, did the orientees like the orientation program? Based on anecdotal feedback from orientees, what could be changed about the orientation program to make it better?

continues

TABLE 6.2 Continued

Learning	What was the measurable difference between pre-orientation and post-orientation tests used to assess cognitive knowledge in caring for adult patients with general medical and surgical problems?
	In a simulated setting, can nurses who have recently completed the orientation program perform the skills required in that unit?
Behavior	In the actual unit, can nurses who have recently completed the orientation program perform the skills required in that unit?
	What progress do preceptors, educators, and/or peers observe in the orientees with respect to clinical skills, decision-making, delegation, etc.?
Results	Did the reduction in orientation length yield the same degree of competency as nurses who completed a longer orientation?
	Do patients report a comparable degree of care received between nurses who recently completed orientation and those who have been working on the unit for an extended period of time?

You may note that many of the examples we used to describe Kirkpatrick's model involved assessing an orientation program rather than an individual's competency. Unfortunately, there is no single model that is widely accepted as the foundation of assessing a nurse's competence (that is, when they have successfully completed orientation). Some of the outcome measures of an orientation program's efficacy may involve nursing behaviors (for example, Kirkpatrick's learning and behavior levels can provide evaluation of an individual's performance). However, a holistic evaluation of an orientee is different from that of the organization, and the former is covered in Chapter 4.

Other Evaluation Models

Additional models (or methods) for evaluation include RSA, CIPP, ROI, and CBR. It may also be appropriate to choose a QI approach. (And you thought you had been in healthcare long enough to know all the abbreviations out there! Let's briefly explore these.)

RSA (Roberta S. Abruzzese)

The RSA Model gets its name from the originator of the model, Roberta S. Abruzzese (1992). Her model is described in Table 6.3. It looks pretty similar to Kirkpatrick's model, right?

TABLE 6.3 *RSA Model Overview*

	DESCRIPTION	EXAMPLES
Process	Known as the "happiness index," this level measures learner satisfaction	Surveys Facilitated Group Discussions
Content	Measures the degree to which knowledge, skills, or attitudes were acquired or changed	Pre-Test/Post-Test Self-Assessments Simulations Case Studies
Outcome	Measures behavioral or performance change after returning to the clinical environment (typically assessed several months after the program)	Self-Assessments Direct Observation
Impact	Measures organizational results	Retention/Turnover Rates Quality Indicators Cost-Benefit Ratios
Total Program	Includes all other components (process, content, outcome, and impact) for a "big picture" view	Annual Reports

Source: Abruzzese (1992)

ROI (Return on Investment) and CBR (Cost-Benefit Ratio)

Determining an ROI or CBR allows you to place dollar signs into your evaluation data, which may speak with greater influence than other evaluation methods (depending on your audience). Both calculations provide similar data, but their formulas are slightly different:

ROI (%) = (Benefits – Costs) / Costs x 100

CBR = (Program Benefits) / (Program Costs)

The goal result in these calculations would be to obtain a number greater than or equal to 100% (for an ROI) or 1 (for a CBR). That would indicate the benefits (return) are greater than the costs (investments). Unfortunately, determining these values may be costly (pun intended). Consider the following two examples:

REAL-WORLD EXAMPLE: USING ROI/CBR IN YOUR EVALUATIONS, EASY EXAMPLE

Beth is a unit-based educator who would like to implement a preceptor training and development program because she believes it will enhance the orientation experience for both preceptors and orientees. She would like to provide a 4-hour class to 10 of her preceptors (who make $25/hour). Additionally, it will cost Beth about $500 in preparing content and developing learning materials. This means the cost of the program is $1,500 for both the preceptors' salaries along with the program development.

If she has a hunch that this could decrease the length of orientation (because the preceptors have gained additional skills), Beth could measure this impact in terms of salary. Let's say each preceptor oriented two nurses during the year, and these orientees had a shorter orientation than the previous year (by an average of two shifts, or 16 hours). If these orientees made $20/hour, that would mean they saved $6,400. Beth could display her results as follows:

ROI = ($6,400 – $1,500) / $1,500 x 100 = 327%

CBR = $6,400 / $1,500 = 4.3

Either way, it is obvious the benefits (return) were well worth the costs (investment).

We call that an easy example because the number of factors to consider for calculation are few. Consider this example that falls on the other end of the spectrum:

REAL-WORLD EXAMPLE: USING ROI/CBR IN YOUR EVALUATIONS, DIFFICULT EXAMPLE

Dena is a unit-based educator who is frustrated with the difficulty orientees experience in constructing complex intravenous line setups in an intensive care unit. She would like to standardize the process among all of the units and create charts and figures the orientees could use as a reference (rather than learning and relearning various approaches from different preceptors—a time-consuming endeavor). To determine an ROI or CBR, Dena will need to consider, at minimum, the following factors in her calculations:

Cost/Investment—Dena's time (salary) spent in meetings with other units and stakeholders, chart/figure development, simulation supplies for teaching the new setup, etc.

Benefit/Return—Decreased time in training, decreased amount of wasted supplies, decreased cost of line infections (if any), etc.

Do you see the difficulty in collecting data in the latter example? Unfortunately, it may not be practical to use this type of evaluation for this particular project. Dena may have to settle for objective data at the satisfaction level only in this case.

QI (Quality Improvement)

QI has recently become a buzz phrase in many organizations as it allows clinicians who have relatively little experience in research to implement change projects rapidly, while ensuring valid statistical analysis of changes in outcome measures. Nursing professional development specialists could consider the use of these methods for evaluating the statistical significance of changes in metrics that are both objective and quantifiable in nature. There are several variations in methodological approaches (for example, Six Sigma or LEAN). Unfortunately, the process for engaging in rigorous QI projects is a bit more complex than we can place in one chapter. If you want more information on these methodologies, we invite you to contact your organization's quality improvement staff or check some of the reliable Internet sites we provide in the nearby sidebar.

KEY QI METHODS

The following are some of the key QI approaches you could choose to implement and where you can go to find more about them:

- *The Institute for Healthcare Improvement is a great resource dedicated to many facets of process and quality improvement within healthcare (http://www.ihi.org/).*
- *Six Sigma focuses on developing highly efficient, standardized processes (http://www.6sigma.us/).*
- *LEAN is similar to Six Sigma but focuses more on reducing and eliminating waste (http://www.lean.org/).*

Summary of Models

It doesn't really matter which evaluation model or method you use as long as you use one that provides a systematic approach to evaluating program efficacy. They are all valid approaches, so you should pick one that makes sense to you, that you enjoy using, and that is practical given the resources you have at your disposal.

Additionally, you don't necessarily need to use every level of evaluation in every program. As you have hopefully seen in the examples, the different levels are more appropriate in different situations, and some levels aren't even feasible in some cases. The goal is to have the greatest number of evaluation levels and/or the levels that demonstrate the greatest impact on patient care, but time and other resources will likely limit the degree to which this can be accomplished.

Evaluating an Organization's Orientation Program

Because we have already listed several examples of applying Kirkpatrick's model to an orientation program, let's now look at the big-picture, organizational view of evaluating an orientation program. As you know, hospitals, clinics, and other organizations come in various shapes and sizes with different infrastructures for a nursing professional development (or nursing education) department. Some organizations have adopted an entirely centralized department, some are completely decentralized, and some have eclectic combinations of the two. Smaller organizations may not even have a dedicated education department, but rather the nurse manager or director is responsible for staff development.

Regardless of the structure in your organization, the following methods and ideas can be modified to meet your needs. Also keep in mind that no one, single path should be considered the "right" way of doing orientation, and the most important consideration in evaluating an orientation program is answering the question, "Does the orientation program meet the needs of the organization while supporting its mission, vision, and values?"

Because we can't directly answer that important question for you, we want to provide you with additional questions that could help you answer that foundational one. Use Worksheet 6.1 to help you evaluate your organization's orientation program through a "define and discover" approach.

WORKSHEET 6.1 *Evaluating an Organization's Orientation Program*

DEFINE ("What is/are...")	DISCOVER ("How is your orientation program...")
...the organization's mission?	...contributing toward the organization achieving its mission?
...the organization's vision?	...helping the organization move toward its vision?
...the organization's values?	...assisting new employees in learning, incorporating, and supporting the values of the organization?
...the organization's greatest needs at this time (e.g., recent sentinel events, poor quality indicators, recommendations from an accrediting body survey, cost reduction, etc.)?	...addressing those needs?
...the principals (key stakeholders) in the organization, and what do they want out of the orientation program?	...meeting their goals and desires?
...other important factors to consider from your Assessment/ Analysis performed in Chapter 2?	...meeting the needs identified in the Assessment/Analysis stage?

continues

WORKSHEET 6.1 *Continued*

DEFINE	DISCOVER
Final Question: Are there any other components currently included in your orientation program that are not listed elsewhere?	**Final Question:** If so, are they still needed, or should you consider removing them?

As you complete Worksheet 6.1, try to think of the outcome measures that will provide the highest level of objective evaluation while also being feasible. Doing this will help you stay on track to provide the principals (stakeholders) with evidence for changing or maintaining an orientation's activities. (It will also help you in preparing for a presentation or writing a publication when you discover a best practice worth sharing with others in the profession!)

Evaluating a Unit's/Department's Orientation Program

Many of the concepts mentioned in evaluating an organization's orientation program also will be applicable to a unit's/department's orientation program. However, the principals at this level may be different, so desired outcome measures may vary. For example, principals at the organizational level may include senior-level managers while principals at the unit/departmental level may include preceptors and even patients.

Therefore, the "define and discover" approach used at this level will be very similar to the one used at the organizational level. However, we thought it was worth placing the worksheet (6.2) here again with modifications already made to make it easier (and quicker!) to use.

WORKSHEET 6.2 *Evaluating an Unit's/Department's Orientation Program*

DEFINE ("What is/are...")	DISCOVER ("How is your orientation program...")
...the unit's/department's mission?	...contributing toward the unit department achieving its mission?

DEFINE	DISCOVER
…the unit's/department's vision?	…helping the unit/department move toward its vision?
…the unit's/department's values?	…assisting new employees in learning, incorporating, and supporting the values of the unit/department?
…the expected behaviors (i.e., competencies) of other staff in the unit/department?	…helping new hires learn those expectations and practice them consistently?
…the unit's/department's greatest needs at this time? (e.g., recent sentinel events, poor quality indicators, recommendations from an accrediting body survey, cost reduction, etc.)	…addressing those needs?
…the principals (key stakeholders) in the unit/department, and what do they want out of the orientation program?	…meeting their goals/desires?
…other important factors to consider from your Assessment/ Analysis as discussed in Chapter 2?	…meeting the needs identified in the Assessment/Analysis stage?
Final Question: Are there any other components currently included in your orientation program that are not listed elsewhere?	**Final Question:** If so, are they still needed, or should you consider removing them?

Evaluating an Individual's Orientation

Many evaluation strategies apply to an individual's orientation, too. The biggest difference will be that the behavior/outcome level (how they are performing in the clinical setting) is probably always being evaluated by a peer, preceptor, or educator and will determine *when* they are done with orientation (if you use a competency-based orientation program). This component is discussed more thoroughly in Chapter 4.

Additionally, unlike many programs in which evaluation is performed at the completion of the program, evaluating an individual's orientation experience will occur both during the process and at its completion.

You want to evaluate an individual's orientation experience for several reasons:

- Individuals may provide more insight into opportunities for improving an orientation program than does aggregated survey data.

- Feedback can be acquired on preceptor performance.

- An individual's experiences during orientation will set the stage for his/her attitude toward his/her work environment, and you have the opportunity to check for any negative attitudes that may have surfaced.

- Evaluating an individual's experience (and making modifications, if required) demonstrates to the employee that you care about him/her as a person.

Following a similar format to the models discussed previously in this chapter, Table 6.4 is a guide to help evaluate an individual's orientation program and experience.

TABLE 6.4 *Evaluating an Individual's Orientation*

COMPONENT	EVALUATION ACTIVITIES
Satisfaction/Reaction/Process	Ask: How was your orientation experience? What did you like or dislike about it?
	Do: Postevaluation Survey with Likert scales as well as open-ended questions
Learning/Content	Ask: What was the best thing you learned in orientation? What were the easiest/hardest things to learn? What are your current strengths and areas for improvement?
	Do: Multiple-Choice Exam(s) assessing basic competencies; Acquire Preceptor Feedback
Behavior/Outcome	Ask: Do you see yourself performing patient care in a safe manner? What are your current strengths and areas for improvement?
	Do: Chart Audits; Direct Observation; Acquire Preceptor Feedback

COMPONENT	EVALUATION ACTIVITIES
Results/Impact	Not Applicable

Note: These questions do not necessarily need to be asked in the past tense. You could (and should) modify these to ask them in present tense while the orientee is currently in orientation, too.

Tools/Handouts

Worksheet 6.3 can be used to help you evaluate your own program. It combines features of several models discussed in this chapter.

WORKSHEET 6.3 *Questions to Guide Program Evaluation*

COMPONENT	QUESTIONS TO ASK
Satisfaction/Reaction/Process	How will you measure learner satisfaction? (surveys, Likert scales, open-ended responses, in-person or group interviews, immediately following program vs. delayed, etc.)
Learning/Content	How will you measure the degree to which knowledge, skills, or attitudes were acquired or changed? (pre-test/post-test exams, case studies, self-report, etc.)
Behavior/Outcome	How will you measure performance while in the clinical setting? (direct observation, self-report, peer assessment, chart audits, etc.)
Results/Impact	How will you measure the unit/organizational impact? (cost [ROI/CBR], patient care [quality indicators or dashboards], etc.)
Already Measuring	Are there any measures currently being assessed in the organization that could relate to your program? (quality indicators, length of orientation, etc.)
Who/When	Who is going to collect the data you would like measured, and when are they going to do it?
Other	What other components should be considered in evaluating this program?

Conclusion

Using a systematic evaluation approach, regardless of what specific model you use, will keep you on track and prevent overlooking an important component of the program. Structured evaluation, especially at higher and/or multiple levels, also demonstrates to others that you have a solid orientation program that wasn't created on a whim.

On a final note, in any organization, there will always be changes in leadership structure and/or new personnel in various decision-making positions. Keeping records of evaluation data will help in telling the story of how programs came to be what they are and prevent new people from "learning the hard way" when they want to try something new. Don't let all your hard work in evaluation go to waste; keep records (at least summaries) of the evaluations you perform.

Questions for Reflection/Discussion

1. What processes do you currently have in place for evaluating your orientation program?

2. Do you feel your current orientation program meets the needs of your unit/department or organization?

3. Could you use additional models or levels of evaluation to more fully demonstrate the efficacy of your orientation program?

4. How do you see the use of multiple evaluation methods assisting you in building a case for additional orientation resources?

5. What processes do you currently have in place for evaluating an individual's orientation experience, and what (if anything) could be done to enhance this evaluation?

KEY TAKEAWAYS

- *Evaluating an organization's, unit's, and individual's onboarding program/experience is vitally important in the continued efficacy of the onboarding process.*
- *Perform evaluations regularly and as close as possible to the end of a program.*
- *Seek feedback from multiple sources.*
- *Multiple models can be used to evaluate an onboarding program, and while each one has its strengths and weaknesses, using a variety of models and levels will likely be the best approach.*

References

Abruzzese, R. S. (1992). *Nursing staff development: Strategies for success.* St. Louis, MO: Mosby.

Kirkpatrick, D. (1996). Great ideas revisited: Revisiting Kirkpatrick's four-level model. *Training and Development, 50*(1), 54–59.

CHAPTER 7

Regulatory Considerations

Introduction

If you've been in nursing for even a short period of time, you're
very aware of the plethora of rules, regulations, governing boards,
accrediting bodies, etc., that set practice standards for what you do as a
nurse. From basic scope of practice standards such as delegation to the
more complex requirements such as annual competency assessments,
external entities play a huge role in ensuring safe patient care. Many
nurses (and especially nurse managers) get antsy at the thought of a visit
from a regulatory body, and there is likely a lot of tension throughout
the organization during a review. It can be easy to think of these
agencies trying to scrutinize every little detail to the point of being just
plain ridiculous.

We want to start this discussion on regulatory issues by changing
the perspective just a little. Rather than looking at a regulatory body's
purpose as attempting to make your life as difficult as possible, try to

see them through a patient's eyes. The regulatory bodies are simply trying to protect patients and their loved ones from poor healthcare practices. And guess what? If you follow the tips we've outlined in this chapter, you'll already have your ducks in a row, and there will be no need to worry about issues during a visit from these agencies.

To help with this, start by recognizing that most regulatory agencies do not tell you *how* to do something but rather *what* you need to do. Take the example of the Joint Commission's requirement for staff training related to caring for patients of different ages. Most nurses are probably aware of this requirement, and many organizations provide a unique, annual age-specific education module to all direct-care providers. However, in looking at the Joint Commission's requirement (at least as it was displayed at the time this book was written), it states that education should be specific to the populations served by the organizations. This could imply that not only should different age groups be included but perhaps also different cultures (which we now know they do include based on subsequent recommendations from the Joint Commission). The other problem with this distinct education module is that the guideline does not require a separate piece of education. You could consider incorporating age and culture-specific information into educational initiatives already occurring (for example, educating on different sizes of restraints, or building case studies that involve patients of different cultures).

The point we're trying to make is that you shouldn't build mountains that you can't climb, so try to integrate as many accrediting body and regulatory requirements as possible into fewer diverse education modules rather than having a separate module for each standard. Table 7.1 gives a quick example of what we mean by combining these modules. The bottom line is that you will find overlapping regulations, requirements, etc., so build them into existing modules where the content makes sense. This will make you and your staff members a lot happier.

In this chapter, we'll cover key concepts related to accrediting bodies, state and federal government mandates, and finally documentation. There will definitely be some overlap in these areas, but Figure 7.1 describes what makes these distinct.

TABLE 7.1 *Two Examples of Combining Multiple Regulatory Requirements Into One Education Module*

MODULE & CONTENT	CONTENT MANDATED BY:	RATIONALE
Safety Curriculum: Employee safety behaviors (e.g., wearing personal protective equipment, cleaning up hazardous materials)	Occupational Safety and Health Administration (OSHA)	Because both of these organizations have expected safety behaviors and goals, you could combine these (and even organizations!) into one module discussing "safety" rather than having two separate modules.
Patient safety goals (e.g., patient identification, healthcare-acquired infections)	The Joint Commission (TJC)	
Restraints Across the Lifespan: Indications, application, and monitoring of restraints for patients of all age groups.	The Joint Commission (TJC) Centers for Medicare & Medicaid Services (CMS)	TJC requires both restraint and population-specific training, while CMS requires restraint training.

> **NOTE**
>
> *Disclaimer: We are not licensed attorneys. In fact, we are not attorneys at all, nor do we play attorneys on television! We are not providing any type of legal or regulatory advice. If you have questions about a certain situation, please contact your nursing leader and/or Human Resources.*

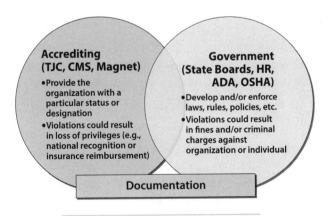

FIGURE 7.1

Distinctions between accrediting and governmental bodies. (Note that documentation's role is to provide evidence to demonstrate compliance with regulatory standards.)

Accreditation Standards

Accrediting bodies are those external organizations that provide a particular credential, certification, or status for an organization based upon the fulfillment of a minimum set of criteria. Different organizations (and even departments) have different accrediting bodies that could set these expectations. For example, the American Nurses Credentialing Center (ANCC) can designate an entire hospital system as achieving Magnet status, while the American Association of Critical-Care Nurses (AACN) could designate an intensive care unit as achieving the Beacon Award for Excellence. The intensive care unit receiving the Beacon award that exists within a hospital system holding a Magnet designation would be responsible for meeting expectations set by both accrediting bodies.

While some of these accrediting bodies are responsible for recognizing excellence (such as the aforementioned Magnet and Beacon recognitions), other accrediting bodies provide certain privileges (for example, the Centers for Medicare and Medicaid Services sets expectations of organizations that wish to receive insurance reimbursement). In contrast to the governmental (legal) issues that follow this section, an organization's participation in the accrediting process is typically voluntary, albeit highly desired. They all contain a wide variety of requirements, but we want to briefly focus on the expectations they set for newly hired employees.

We do not wish to provide an exhaustive list of expectations from each of these organizations for two reasons:

1. The organizations can change their expectations at any time, so it is best for you to find the most current guidelines.

2. Each organization may interpret the guidelines slightly differently.

Most organizations make their accrediting manuals available to employees. If you don't know where to find a particular manual, contact your manager or compliance officer for additional information. Once you find the source manual, search through it looking for words like *orientation, training, initial, competency,* and *hire.* As you find these, write those statements down and begin building a list of things that must be included. Once you extract these statements from all the agencies to which you report, you will have all the necessary guidelines to ensure you can withstand an audit (as long as you also implement their requests and document performance of them). Although this might sound like a lot, you'll probably quickly find that many of the external agencies have quite a bit of overlap (such as waived testing or restraint requirements).

The Joint Commission

If you work in a hospital, home care, or behavioral health, you are well aware of the Joint Commission (TJC) and its many requirements. Because this likely will apply to the majority of readers, we will use this accrediting body as an example. However, many other accrediting bodies are specific to smaller organizations, such as college health clinics and ambulatory surgery centers (Accreditation Association for Ambulatory Health Care), community health centers (Community Health Accreditation Program), and so on. Accreditation by these organizations designates your facility as an organization where patients can expect to receive high-quality care. Because of this, many of the organizations focus on active improvement work (in addition to meeting basic requirements) to continue pushing the envelope on what is considered quality care.

Regarding orientation, TJC outlines several requirements as being necessary. One of the most basic requirements is simply that the organization provides an orientation to staff. TJC offers a few specifics of what must be included in that orientation, but there is also a lot of freedom in what can be included. Typically, their guidelines ask that you train new personnel in the following specific areas and document successful completion of the training (TJC, 2013):

- Basic job duties
- Pain management
- Cultural diversity
- Patient rights and ethical issues
- Performing waived tests
- Restraints

Centers for Medicare and Medicaid Services

Similar to TJC, the Centers for Medicare and Medicaid Services (CMS) sets minimum expectations; however, CMS does not require the degree of improvement work that TJC does. Instead, CMS sets Conditions of Participation (CoP), which are minimum requirements that must be met to receive reimbursement for patients using Medicare or Medicaid. If these CoPs are not met, the organization risks losing its major funding source, as other insurance companies will also cease reimbursement activities to follow suit with CMS.

With respect to orientation, CMS requires documentation of the following nonexhaustive items (CMS, 2012):

- Initial training and competency assessment
- Abuse and neglect
- Blood and blood product administration
- Medication preparation and administration
- Restraints and seclusion

In addition to basic requirements for various organizations (for example, hospitals have specific criteria), some programs within organizations have additional requirements (for example, if hospitals manage patients receiving solid organ transplants, transplant-specific criteria will also be required of the hospital).

Other Regulatory Bodies

In addition to these major accrediting bodies, other agencies may also regulate activities at your organization. For example, the American Association of Blood Banks (AABB) will regulate all activities surrounding storage, handling, and administration of blood and blood products. You would be wise to review the orientation expectations of these organizations as well; however, you will likely note significant overlap between their orientation-specific guidelines and those of CMS and TJC. Ancillary regulatory bodies to consider may include:

- American Association of Blood Banks (AABB)
- College of American Pathologists (CAP)

- Commission on the Accreditation of Rehabilitation Facilities (CARF)

- American College of Surgeons, Commission on Cancer (CoC)

The only difference may be excellence awards (like the American Nurses Credentialing Center's [ANCC] Magnet designation) that designate organizations as achieving more than the minimum standards. Requirements for these external agencies will be much higher than other regulatory bodies.

Government (Legal) Issues

Once again, working with accrediting bodies is a voluntary process to receive a designation associated with privileges. In contrast, government (legal) issues are mandatory. We want to share some legal concerns with you that relate to the orientation and onboarding process of new employees. These include:

- Licensure and certification

- Employment laws

- Occupational safety standards

- Working with your Human Resources department.

Licensure and Certification

Many people get the terms *license* and *certificate* confused.

- A license is a government-issued document that allows you to perform certain tasks once you meet certain qualifications. Take a driver's *license* for example. A driver's license is issued from the state government where you are a resident once you have passed a written and driving exam. Once you have the license, you are permitted to operate certain vehicles. Similarly, a nursing *license* is issued by the state's board of nursing to individuals who have received an academic nursing degree and passed a national exam.

- A certificate is offered by governmental or nongovernmental entities and recognizes additional accomplishment or an expanded scope of practice beyond licensure. For example, additional accomplishment is demonstrated when a public health nurse has worked in a public health setting for a certain number of hours and passes a national exam. The nurse still maintains his/her same licensure but is now also certified.

Regarding scope of practice expansion, many states do not provide a nurse practitioner *license* but rather a *certificate*. In those states, nurse practitioners still practice under their RN licenses.

Licensure is required for independently caring for patients as an RN (and in many situations, even before starting orientation); certification is not. Someone in the organization should be verifying licensure through methods appropriate for that state. This is known as primary source verification and is more commonly being performed online.

During a new hire's orientation and onboarding process, the new employee should be exposed to the appropriate scope of practice for that state. You should be able to easily access the nurse practice act for your state to assist the new employee with this. You may also want to be aware of some components of the practice acts from the board of medicine and board of pharmacy to help illustrate what is *outside* the scope of practice for a nurse.

Key Employment Laws That Impact Onboarding

Several key employment laws could impact your new nurse's onboarding process. They include:

- Americans with Disabilities Act (ADA)
- Family and Medical Leave Act (FMLA)
- Pregnancy Discrimination Act (PDA)
- Title VII of the Civil Rights Act (Title VII)
- Fair Labor Standards Act (FLSA)

Let's look at these one at a time.

Americans with Disabilities Act (ADA)

The American with Disabilities Act (ADA) protects people with disabilities, those perceived to have disabilities, as well as employees who are associated with someone with disabilities (U.S. Equal Employment Opportunity Commission, 2013b). The U.S. Equal Employment Opportunity Commission (EEOC) oversees violations of the ADA. The EEOC has a special page designated for the ADA and healthcare workers. We suggest that you look at http://www.eeoc.gov/facts/health_care_workers.html for more information.

So, how does ADA impact you with your new employees? Well, there could be several ways. Consider these potential scenarios.

REAL-WORLD EXAMPLE: ADA SCENARIO #1

Jolene has been hired and tells you right away that she has vision issues and requires reasonable accommodation. What do you do?

1. *First, ensure that the hiring manager and Human Resources were aware of the issue before Jolene was hired.*
2. *Second, have Human Resources determine what Jolene needs in terms of reasonable accommodation.*
3. *Third, evaluate Jolene working with her reasonable accommodation as you would any other new nurse.*

Jolene is working the night shift on a unit where the modus operandi is to leave the overhead lights off when checking on patients. Jolene is accommodated with a flashlight that allows her to check vitals, etc., without disturbing the patient with overhead lights.

REAL-WORLD EXAMPLE: ADA SCENARIO #2

Fred starts onboarding and you notice that he seems to have difficulty hearing patients, their families, and you. This concerns you because you also notice that he is challenged when listening for respiration and heart sounds. What do you do?

1. *First, talk with Fred and see if he mentions any hearing issues.*
2. *Regardless of his answer, talk with his hiring manager and Human Resources next. Explain your concerns to them and tell them about the conversation with Fred.*
3. *Third, Human Resources and the hiring manager should meet with Fred to discuss the issue.*

continues

It appears that Fred does have some hearing difficulties, but not to the level of being considered hearing disabled. That said, since it is perceived that his hearing challenge impacts his ability to do his work, a reasonable accommodation should be made, as the ADA requires accommodations for people who are perceived to be disabled. A special stethoscope is provided for Fred, and you notice that his ability to hear respiration and heart sounds improves. Things seem to be improving, until several members from different patients' families complain that they have to repeat everything three or four times with Fred. One time, he brought the wrong pain medicine to a patient because he didn't hear clearly.

At this point, you work to determine whether Fred (a) understands what medicines can be used for pain or (b) did not hear the patient. You may administer a pain medication test. He passes the test, so you document that he has the cognitive knowledge. Take the situation and results to the hiring manager and Human Resources. They will determine Fred's employment status.

What are the key takeaways from these examples? First, the ADA requires that reasonable accommodations be made so that differently-abled people can do their jobs. Second, once the reasonable accommodation is provided, the person must still be able to do all the activities of the job in a safe manner. Finally, when in doubt, bring issues to the attention of the hiring manager and your Human Resources specialist.

Family and Medical Leave Act (FMLA)

The Family and Medical Leave Act (FMLA) "entitles eligible employees of covered employers to take unpaid, job-protected leave for specified family and medical reasons with continuation of group health insurance coverage under the same terms and conditions as if the employee had not taken leave. Eligible employees are entitled to:

"Twelve workweeks of leave in a 12-month period for:

- the birth of a child and to care for the newborn child within one year of birth;

- the placement with the employee of a child for adoption or foster care and to care for the newly placed child within one year of placement;

- to care for the employee's spouse, child, or parent who has a serious health condition;

- a serious health condition that makes the employee unable to perform the essential functions of his or her job;

- any qualifying exigency arising out of the fact that the employee's spouse, son, daughter, or parent is a covered military member on 'covered active duty;' or

"Twenty-six workweeks of leave during a single 12-month period to care for a covered service member with a serious injury or illness if the eligible employee is the service member's spouse, son, daughter, parent, or next of kin (military caregiver leave)" (U.S. Department of Labor, 2013d).

What's the potential impact of FMLA and your new nurses? Let's take a look at a couple scenarios.

REAL-WORLD EXAMPLE: FMLA SCENARIO #1

Jeremy's partner has been diagnosed with metastatic breast cancer. She will require surgery, chemo, and reconstruction. Jeremy talks with his hiring manager and Human Resources and applies for intermittent FMLA. Unfortunately, Jeremy misses an important class on new regulations because of his partner's illness. What do you do?

Before Jeremy leaves the day before his partner's surgery, tell him, "Jeremy, I wish you and your partner the best tomorrow. Please keep us posted on her progress. You probably saw that tomorrow, we are holding a class on new regulations. Don't worry about it. As soon as you get back to the unit, I'll review the new regs with you and make sure you understand how they impact our work."

Some organizations will record these sessions so that employees who are unable to attend can still get the information. If that is not possible, work with Jeremy the next time he is present to ensure that he understands the new regulations and how they impact work on the unit.

REAL-WORLD EXAMPLE: FMLA SCENARIO #2

Reva has been missing work, and you notice that it seems to be mostly Mondays and Fridays. You hear from her friend that Reva's dad is quite ill, and she's been going to her hometown on weekends to relieve her mom.

continues

Obviously, you are concerned about Reva and her family...and her ability to complete the onboarding. What do you do?

Talk with Reva. Say, "Reva, I've noticed that you've been missing work, mostly on Mondays and Fridays. Is there something going on that I should know about?" Reva tells you and seems relieved to have told someone else at work.

You say, "Let's go talk with your manager. You and she should talk with HR about the Family and Medical Leave Act and how you can best support your family during this difficult time, as well as protect your employment."

FMLA can be challenging to manage, especially when you are trying to get an orientee ready to go solo in your unit; however, remember that it is important for the orientee to know that his or her loved one is getting the medical treatment and support he or she needs. Communication during this time is critical so that you know when the orientee is available for additional training. The orientee will work with his or her manager regarding scheduled days away, reporting that time, etc. Your focus should be making good use of the time when the orientee is available.

Pregnancy Discrimination Act (PDA)

According to the U.S. Equal Employment Opportunity Commission, "The Pregnancy Discrimination Act (PDA) forbids discrimination based on pregnancy when it comes to any aspect of employment, including hiring, firing, pay, job assignments, promotions, layoff, training, fringe benefits, such as leave and health insurance, and any other term or condition of employment" (EEOC, 2013a).

A pregnant employee's situation may warrant coverage under ADA as well as FMLA. If you have a pregnant employee in onboarding, work closely with the hiring manager and Human Resources to ensure that you are compliant with the relevant laws. For new employees (and especially those who are new graduate nurses) who must stop their orientation and onboarding process for a period of time, it may be difficult to pick up right where they left off. Therefore, to provide these employees with an effective learning experience while also staying in compliance with federal mandates, you may want to extend their total time spent in orientation to account for this abrupt pause in the learning experience.

REAL-WORLD EXAMPLE: PDA SCENARIO #1

Chelsea is 6 months into her pregnancy when she develops preeclampsia. She tells you that her doctor has provided written documentation requesting light duty for her. What do you do?

You should talk with the hiring manager and Human Resources to ensure that Chelsea has provided the proper documentation. Her hiring manager then meets with her and explains that due to her medical situation, her onboarding will be suspended so that she can be on "light" duty, and her onboarding will continue when she returns from her maternity leave. "Light" duty for someone in the onboarding phase could involve finishing any additional classes or modules necessary for completing orientation, or even performing audits or other administrative work on the unit, which could even be beneficial from a socialization perspective with her peers.

REAL-WORLD EXAMPLE: PDA SCENARIO #2

Rachel is 8 months pregnant, and her water breaks on shift. You get her over to labor and delivery and call her partner. Rachel is 4 weeks into her onboarding process. What do you do?

You buy flowers and a teddy bear and deliver them to her room! Actually, you notify her hiring manager and Human Resources. Hopefully, Rachel has filed all the necessary paperwork for her maternity leave.

Again, communication is critical. As long as the orientee is able, work the program as you would normally. When the orientee is not able, work with the hiring manager and Human Resources specialist to make the appropriate changes in duty or schedule. Finally, when the orientee returns from maternity leave, provide some time for review before getting the orientee back into full orientation mode.

Title VII of the Civil Rights Act (Title VII)

The Civil Rights Act of 1964 is a seminal piece of legislation. Title VII of that act provided for protection against discrimination due to race, color, religion, sex, or national origin. Based on additional legislation, discrimination based on age, pregnancy status, and disabilities is also prohibited (EEOC, 2013b). Check http://www.eeoc.gov/laws/statutes/titlevii.cfm for more information. In general, Title VII should not be a factor, because the law and your organization prohibit discrimination based on the categories listed, and your organization may include other categories such as sexual orientation and/or gender identity. Let's look at a quick scenario under which Title VII would be applicable.

REAL-WORLD EXAMPLE: TITLE VII SCENARIO

Abdullah is a new nurse. On your first day together, he mentions that he is Muslim and needs to pray several times during his shift. What do you do?

You check with Human Resources and find a private room where Abdullah can bring his prayer mat and pray. You ask him to find you when he has finished with his prayers and then continue the onboarding process. If the timing of the prayers may have a negative impact on patient care, discussions with the employee, hiring manager, and Human Resources should be held promptly.

Fair Labor Standards Act (FLSA)

The Fair Labor Standards Act (FLSA) "establishes minimum wage, overtime pay, recordkeeping, and youth employment standards affecting employees in the private sector and in Federal, State, and local governments. Covered nonexempt workers are entitled to a minimum wage of not less than $7.25 per hour effective July 24, 2009. Overtime pay at a rate not less than one and one-half times the regular rate of pay is required after 40 hours of work in a workweek" (U.S. Department of Labor, 2013c).

So, how does this affect you when onboarding new nurses? The main concern regarding FLSA is ensuring that an hourly employee is paid for any and all time worked, and his/her time must be reported in accordance with your organization's policies.

REAL-WORLD EXAMPLE: FLSA SCENARIO

Shelby is a new nurse. You have kept her busy during the shift, and it's time for her to go home. She tells you that she's going to log in to the hospital's intranet from home and complete some regulations training tonight. What do you do?

You say, "Shelby, it's OK to look on the intranet for your schedule, but it is against hospital policy for you to complete training at home."

Shelby responds, "Why? That seems silly."

You say, "Well, because the training is mandatory, we are required by law to pay you for your time. Our policy states that you cannot work from home."

Occupational Safety and Health Administration

The Occupational Safety and Health Administration (OSHA) is a government entity that is responsible for ensuring employees are able to work in safe and healthy environments. For healthcare workers, this will include items such as blood-borne pathogen exposure, respiratory illness protection, and hazardous waste management (U.S. Department of Labor, 2013b). All new employees (not just nurses) will need safety/health training upon hire, and we recommend contacting your Human Resources department to explore what is already being covered in general orientation. If you are part of a smaller organization, you can refer directly to OSHA's website (http://www.osha.gov), as it contains many training resources for you.

Working With Human Resources

You may have noticed that Human Resources comes up a lot in this chapter. How can you best work with your Human Resources person? As a 20-year veteran of HR, Robin has a few tips. Before we start the list, the main thing to remember is that your Human Resources professional's goal is to help you, the orientee, the hiring manager, and the organization be successful. Your HR person can partner with you on hiring, orienting, retaining, disciplining, and many other situations that arise with employees. We recommend that you:

- Develop a good relationship with your Human Resources person.
- When in doubt, contact the hiring manager and Human Resources.
- Stay current on your organization's HR policies and procedures.
- Become briefly familiar with the laws and regulations laid out in this chapter. (Who knows, you might even be able to impress your friends in HR if you throw around some of their abbreviations?)

Documentation

We couldn't consider this text complete without a proper discussion of every healthcare provider's favorite part of his/her job—documentation (can you hear the sarcasm there?). Documentation of the orientation experience is important from both a regulatory perspective (to prove that all employees have had appropriate training) as well as an organizational quality perspective (to evaluate what works and doesn't work within the organization).

To illustrate its importance, consider the following two scenarios:

REAL-WORLD EXAMPLE: THE IMPORTANCE OF DOCUMENTATION #1

A major error has occurred in which a surgical patient received the procedure on the incorrect limb. The state's health department has been contacted to investigate the situation and wants to review whether or not all employees in the operating room have been properly trained on ensuring the correct surgical site is marked.

The unit-based educators bring spreadsheets with completion dates of all regulatory and accrediting body mandatory education requirements. The auditors can verify that staff members have received the appropriate training, and further exploration of the error can continue.

REAL-WORLD EXAMPLE: THE IMPORTANCE OF DOCUMENTATION #2

Senior level management is looking to reduce orientation length as a means for alleviating financial challenges. They have requested information regarding the average length of the current competency-based orientation. After unit-based educators retrieved orientation documentation over the last 2 years, the educators were able to provide data to management that indicated the current length is well below that of surrounding organizations and requested that orientation length not be cut. Management moved their attention to other areas to enact budget cuts.

In both scenarios, having documentation available provided evidence that the standard was being met. Without this documented data, it can be difficult (or even impossible) to demonstrate compliance and/or performance.

ESSENTIAL DOCUMENTATION

It can be difficult to determine which documents to keep and which ones to trash if you're new to the realm of orientation. To be safe, it is wise to keep more than you trash in the beginning. You can always do some "spring cleaning" once you have a better grasp on what documents are important. To help you get started, though, here are some essential documents we recommend you keep:

- *Offer letter*
- *A copy of licenses and certifications (if these cannot be immediately accessible online)*
- *Proof of orientation completion with signatures of key personnel*
- *Proof of regulatory/mandatory module and class completions*
- *Orientation schedule (along with assigned preceptor)*
- *Rental equipment/supply agreement forms (e.g., pagers, keys)*

Dos and Don'ts

To provide you with some quick action items on how to handle documentation issues, check out Table 7.2, Dos and Don'ts of Orientation Documentation. Rationale for many of these items may be found throughout the chapter.

TABLE 7.2 *Dos and Don'ts of Orientation Documentation*

DO	DON'T
Have all key principals (manager, educator, preceptor, & orientee) sign competency documents.	Don't forget the orientees (they must verify that they have ownership of the learning process, too, and that they acknowledge receipt of all necessary learning opportunities).
Ensure the documents are easily retrievable by the appropriate personnel (managers, auditors, etc.).	Don't neglect security & confidentiality of documents to the degree that anybody could access the records.
Keep proof of initial competency assessment.	Don't keep everything unless it can be easily stored electronically.
Maintain organized records by either alphabetical order or date of hire.	Don't simply throw everything in a pile or closet (if you do, being audited will be a nightmare).

continues

TABLE 7.2 *Continued*

DO	DON'T
Include proof of all regulatory training requirements, especially those mandates ending with the statement "upon hire" (or the like).	Don't depend on the orientee nor one single person or department to keep this record (tracking at both the organizational level and the departmental level may prove beneficial).

Formatting and Medium

To our knowledge, there is no external agency that regulates what the training documents should look like. The formatting of the document and whether it is electronic or on paper is left at the discretion of each organization. As long as the documentation is easily retrievable during an audit and the manager (or his/her designee) can walk an auditor through the document, you are in good shape.

Paper documents are easier to develop and share among preceptors; however, retrieval of data can become more cumbersome (either during an audit or if the nurse transfers to a different unit in the organization where the paperwork looks different). Ornate electronic forms of documentation may not be possible in organizations with limited resources, but even relatively simple documents can be prepared with either Microsoft Word or Microsoft Excel. The benefits of these electronic forms of documentation are that they are easily searchable, and they can be shared and stored with multiple persons. If you work in a very large organization, check with the central learning and development (education) department. It may have a learning management system (LMS) that will make it easier to track your orientees' information as well as provide necessary reports for governing and accrediting bodies.

In regard to format of the document, we want to share one example Alvin helped develop at Cincinnati Children's Hospital Medical Center. This form (Figure 7.2, shown on pages 157–161) is a document used throughout the organization that can be modified by each individual unit/department. The template was developed by the hospital and based on Patricia Benner's Novice to Expert spectrum, the AACN Synergy Model, and the organization's job standards and clinical ladder.

Cincinnati Children's Hospital Medical Center
Department of Patient Services Nursing Services Orientation
Core Competency Assessment Tool for Newly Hired RN's 2013

Name:
Unit:
Educator:
Preceptor:

Phases of Orientation

The 4 phases of orientation, based on Patricia's Benner's novice to expert model, defines increasing complexity of learning, and incorporates the three domains of learning and skill acquisition (cognitive learning, psychomotor skill demonstration, and affective reasoning). The increasing complexity is noted in the expected behaviors supporting each competency statement and phase.

The phases of orientation Is a behavior based approach. It provides that the nurse may progress through orientation based on assessment of demonstrated expected behaviors ensuring competent practice rather than solely on time.

The newly hired RN progresses through orientation with Preceptor Assistance, Preceptor Guidance and then to independent practice with Preceptor as Resource.

Requires manager, educator, preceptor and orientee to meet and sign off as each phase is completed.

Phase I: Weeks 1 and 2 of Orientation   (Education Consultant/Orientation Facilitator Guided)

Phase II: Assimilation   (Preceptor Assistance)
Preceptor is present and actively supports orientee with learning opportunities.
Preceptor teaches and assesses practice of new orientee.

Phase III: Adaptation   (Preceptor Guidance)
Preceptor facilitates learning; maximizes learning opportunities.
Preceptor encourages orientee to identify learning needs.

Phase IV: Synthesis   (Preceptor as a Resource)
Preceptor familiar with orientee's experiences and is available as a resource when needed.

Cincinnati Children's Hospital Medical Center
Department of Patient Services Nursing Services Orientation
Core Competency Assessment Tool for Newly Hired RN's 2013

Name:
Unit:
Educator:
Preceptor:

Environment of Care: Socialization to Unit Environment

Introduce the orientee to the team and key resource people on the unit. Use huddle and rounds as opportunities for the orientee to understand how the team works together on your unit. Make sure that the new staff member learns not only about the layout of the unit but also the unit culture. Set up times to meet on a regular basis. Include the educator and manager at least every 2 weeks. Create an environment where the orientee feels safe to ask questions or express concerns.

Validation Statement	Verification/Source of Evaluation
☐ Demonstrates familiarity with unit resources.	Supported by:
☐ Demonstrates awareness of emergency preparedness resources.	☐ Completion of Learning Opportunities
☐ Demonstrates awareness of parent and guest support services.	

Opportunities		
Introduction to Roles and Responsibilities *HealthCare Team Members* ☐ Director/Managers ☐ Charge RN ☐ RNs ☐ PCA ☐ HUC ☐ Care Coordinator ☐ Educator ☐ Environmental Care	**Finding your way** ☐ Breakroom, restrooms, lockers ☐ Medication room/medication refrigerator ☐ Huddle Room ☐ Child life ☐ Tub/shower room ☐ Kitchen ☐ Dirty utility room ☐ Dirty tube system	**Parent/Guest Support Services** ☐ Laundry Facilities ☐ Parent Meals ☐ Family /Visitor Guidelines ☐ Family Relations **Introduction to unit specific Guidelines/Resources** ☐ Staffing guidelines ☐ Scheduling process ☐ Holiday requirements/rotation

Cincinnati Children's Hospital Medical Center
Department of Patient Services Nursing Services Orientation
Core Competency Assessment Tool for Newly Hired RN's 2013

Name:
Unit:
Educator:
Preceptor:

NURSING PROCESS   Validation Statements

Phase II Assimilation	Phase III Adaptation	Phase IV Synthesis
Demonstrates initial competence in development and use of the *NURSING PROCESS*	Demonstrates development and use of the *NURSING PROCESS*	Demonstrates independent development and use of the *NURSING PROCESS*
Completes appropriate assessment for each Body System. □ Respiratory; Cardiovascular; Endocrine; Genitourinary; Gastrointestinal/Nutritional Status; Head, Ear, Eye, Nose and Throat (HEENT); Integumentary; Musculoskeletal; Neuro/Psychiatric; Reproductive □ Correlates assessment findings from patient care equipment with the physical assessment findings/clinical picture. Treats the patient, not the machine. □ Identifies normal/abnormal findings (Physical, diagnostic testing, vital signs, I&O's, psychosocial and discusses that information with the preceptor.	□ Incorporate the nursing process; prioritize care based upon an assessment continuum. □ Create a plan of care integrating all aspects of clinical findings and assessments. □ Perform admissions, transfers, and/or discharges with preceptor guidance. □ Apply growth and development concepts, cultural considerations and psychosocial needs for patients and families throughout the nursing process. □ Demonstrate ability to locate CCHMC/department resources related to nursing interventions.	□ Consistent use of the nursing process; prioritizes care based upon an assessment continuum. □ Anticipate potential problems and identify potential solutions. □ Independently perform admissions, transfers, and/or discharges. □ Consistently apply growth and development concepts, cultural considerations and psychosocial needs for patients and families. □ Utilize appropriate resources related to nursing interventions. □ Evaluate performance management RN job responsibilities.

Cincinnati Children's Hospital Medical Center
Department of Patient Services Nursing Services Orientation
Core Competency Assessment Tool for Newly Hired RN's 2013

Name:
Unit:
Educator:
Preceptor:

Learning Opportunities for *NURSING PROCESS*

Assessment/Evaluation
- □ Care for __ number of types of patients specific to unit/clinic subspecialty population.
- □ Participates in admission/discharge transfer process
- □ Standard Precautions / Isolation Precautions/PPE
- □ Rounds /huddles
- □ Fall Risk Assessment
- □ Pain Assessment
- □ Catheter Associated Urinary Tract Infection Prevention Bundle CA-UTI
- □ PIV Catheter Care and IV Assessment
- □ CVC and PIV Extravasation and Grading
- □ Situational Awareness (e.g. watcher, family concern, PEWS)
- □ Vital signs
- □ Adult Patient Care

Emergency Care
- □ Change of Shift Bedside Safety Check
- □ Suction Equipment (presence & set up)
- □ Portable Suction
- □ Oxygen Set Up
- □ Portable Oxygen Cylinders
- □ Code Button / Panic Button / Staff Assist
- □ Code Sheets
- □ Call light functions
- □ Crash Cart/Defibrillator
- □ Safe environment (e.g. bed placement, side rails up, nurse server locked)

Equipment/Devices
Patient Monitor
- □ Dash®
- □ Solar®

CCHMC Resource: Equipment How-To & JIT aids (Mosby)
Oxygen Delivery Methods
- □ Nasal Cannula
- □ Simple Mask

Anthropometrics
- □ Standing Scale
- □ Infant Scale

Cincinnati Children's Hospital Medical Center
Department of Patient Services Nursing Services Orientation
Core Competency Assessment Tool for Newly Hired RN's 2013

Name:
Unit:
Educator:
Preceptor:

Notes on Progress Page: This page can be used for documentation by preceptor, educator, and a peer for "just in time" Learning opportunities that the newly hired RN experiences day to day. Notes can include Number of patients assigned /ages of patient / diagnosis / skills and procedures / equipment and devices etc.
In addition, the newly hired RN must be aware of resources and demonstrate ability to access resources in the face of uncertainty. Documentation of examples of how the newly hired RN demonstrates expected Safety behaviors and supporting techniques can be captured on the Notes Progress page.

Preceptor Initials / Date:	Age of Pt:	Type of Pt / Diagnosis:
Notes on Demonstrated Safety Behaviors/ Skills Performed / Equipment Training:		

Preceptor Initials / Date:	Age of Pt:	Type of Pt / Diagnosis:
Notes on Demonstrated Safety Behaviors/ Skills Performed / Equipment Training:		

Cincinnati Children's Hospital Medical Center
Department of Patient Services Nursing Services Orientation
Core Competency Assessment Tool for Newly Hired RN's 2013

Name:
Unit:
Educator:
Preceptor:

Orientation Guideline Phases Completion

Phase II
☐ The components of Phase II are either complete or have been addressed by the preceptor and orientee.
Preceptor Signature: _____   Date: _____
Educator signature: _____   Date: _____
Manager/Director signature: _____   Date: _____

Phase III
☐ The components of Phase III are either complete or have been addressed by the preceptor and orientee.
Preceptor Signature: _____   Date: _____
Educator signature: _____   Date: _____
Manager/Director signature: _____   Date: _____

Phase IV
☐ The components of Phase IV are either complete or have been addressed by the preceptor and orientee.
Preceptor Signature: _____   Date: _____
Educator signature: _____   Date: _____
Manager/Director signature: _____   Date: _____
Orientee signature: _____   Date: _____

Verification/Source of Evaluation
Supported by:
☐ *Completion of Learning Opportunities*

☐ *Skills Checklist*

☐ *Module with Post Test*

Verified by:
☐ *Evidence of Daily Practice*

☐ *Peer/preceptor Assessment*

☐ *Educator Assessment*

☐ *Documentation Review*

Comments:

FIGURE 7.2
Example of a competency document.

What to Keep, Where to Keep It, and How Long to Keep It

Determining what documents to keep can be very overwhelming, especially for new educators and managers. There is a tendency to keep too many things when first starting in the new position to make sure you have all your bases covered. If you start your process by looking up all the appropriate regulatory guidelines and keep track of what they request be documented, you'll be in good shape. Try to place yourself in their shoes and ask yourself, "If I were the auditor, what would I need to see to ensure the organization has provided appropriate training of all new employees in [insert topic: for example, restraints]?"

To help with this, consider attaching the source statement of a regulatory requirement to your competency assessment spreadsheet so that others will know *why* you are tracking certain items. In organizations where nurse leaders frequently change positions, it can be helpful for incoming leaders to see the source statement of a requirement rather than depending on anecdotal stories.

Regarding location of orientation competency documentation, the unit educator may be able to keep documents in his/her office throughout the orientation and onboarding period. Once the new employee has completed the onboarding process (or if a regulatory body performs an audit), all documents should be sent to the manager, who can then forward necessary documents to Human Resources. The reason the manager should have the most easy access to the documents is because the manager (or his/her designee) is the one ultimately responsible for competency assessment, according to most regulatory bodies.

Evidence of initial competency assessment should probably be retained for the duration of an individual's employment in that unit or department. For more general topics (such as patient rights, cultural diversity, etc.), completion documentation should be retained throughout the individual's employment with the organization. Ongoing competency assessment can be destroyed after 3 to 6 years (depending on the particular regulatory body's requirements); however, initial competency records should be retained. This does not necessarily mean that, for example, a 10-page medication quiz must be retained in the employee's record; however, evidence of taking the quiz and passing it (perhaps along with the score) should be placed in writing in the orientation record. Compiling all orientation-related documentation into one folder to place into the employee's personnel file will help keep that record organized and easily retrievable.

Confidentiality

Orientation records, like other personnel records, should remain as confidential as possible. Especially if there were issues during an employee's orientation period that could result in embarrassment for the individual, confidentiality of information should be protected. The manager, orientee, and Human Resources personnel should be the only employees with unlimited access to the personnel record.

Educators likely will have access to most of the orientation record. An exception would be the example of an orientee who must take a medical leave during the orientation period. The manager and Human Resources can work with the orientee on the reason for the leave, but the educator only needs to know when the leave will occur so that scheduling of appropriate learning activities can occur. The orientee is able to share this information with the educator, if desired, but the educator does not *need* access to this information to carry out his/her duties.

Preceptors will need access to a significant portion of the orientation records to carry out their teaching duties. For example, they may need to see preferred learning styles, learning activities already completed, and areas for improvement. They will not need as much access as the educator and manager, but it will be important to keep them in the loop if they are to create a highly effective learning atmosphere.

Other than the orientee, manager, Human Resources, educator, and preceptors, no other employees should need access to information found in the new employee's orientation record. Protecting this information through the use of physical locks or password-protected files will be beneficial in guaranteeing employee privacy and offsetting organizational liability.

NOTE

Regarding documentation, confidentiality, etc.—when in doubt, check with the hiring manager and your Human Resources professional.

Conclusion

The abundance of accrediting and legal guidelines can be quite overwhelming, especially if you don't have much time to explore them on your own. However, the time spent retrieving source statements and becoming familiar with what's actually required will yield a significant return on your investment. We highly recommend taking a day or two to become familiar with all the various requirements and organizing them for yourself. If you can organize the orientation-related requirements and document compliance with all of them, when the auditors come around, you'll have no reason for anxiety.

Questions for Reflection/Discussion

1. What are your greatest fears or challenges regarding regulatory or accrediting bodies?

2. What are possible action steps you could take to become more prepared for a regulatory body or accrediting body audit?

3. What are the strengths and weaknesses of your current approach to documentation of orientation competency assessment?

KEY TAKEAWAYS

- *As healthcare workers, you must stay current on relevant regulatory changes.*
- *Since you are working with orientees, you must stay current on relevant labor laws as well.*
- *Recordkeeping is important to your success and the continued compliance of your organization.*
- *When in doubt, contact your Human Resources liaison.*

References

Centers for Medicare and Medicaid Services (CMS). (2012). State operations manual. Retrieved from http://www.cms.gov/Regulations-and-Guidance/Guidance/Manuals/downloads/som107ap_a_hospitals.pdf

The Joint Commission. (2013). The Joint Commission Manual, E-dition, Release 5.1. Retrieved from http://www.jointcommission.org/

U.S. Department of Labor (2013a). Disability resources, American with Disabilities Act. Retrieved from http://www.dol.gov/dol/topic/disability/ada.htm

U.S. Department of Labor (2013b). Occupational Safety and Health Administration, Clinicians. Retrieved from https://www.osha.gov/dts/oom/clinicians/index.html

U.S. Department of Labor (2013c). Wage and Hour Division (WHD), Compliance assistance—Wages and the Fair Labor Standards Act (FLSA). Retrieved from http://www.dol.gov/whd/flsa/

U.S. Department of Labor (2013d). Wage and Hour Division (WHD), Family and Medical Leave Act. Retrieved from http://www.dol.gov/whd/fmla/

U.S. Equal Employment Opportunity Commission (EEOC). (2013a). Pregnancy discrimination. Retrieved from http://www.eeoc.gov/laws/types/pregnancy.cfm

U.S. Equal Employment Opportunity Commission (EEOC) (2013b). Title VII of the Civil Rights Act of 1964. Retrieved from http://www.eeoc.gov/laws/statutes/titlevii.cfm

CHAPTER 8

Practical Tips for
Staying Organized

Introduction

We hope you've found all the previous content helpful and insightful, but if you're new to managing orientation and onboarding programs, we expect you might be feeling a little overwhelmed at this point. You might even be thinking, "I don't care about improving the system. I just need to be able to keep my head above water!" This chapter is devoted to offering practical tips and examples of how to stay organized.

Why are we devoting a whole chapter to such a basic concept? Well, there are several reasons. Alvin's experience in training new educators has been that even though they have lots of great ideas and enthusiasm, those can quickly be stifled once the number of responsibilities and tasks pile up into a seemingly insurmountable challenge. Additionally, nursing school taught you how to organize patient care, but there was probably no mention of how to organize your office schedule or your email inbox. And, if you are the first professional development specialist your unit has had, there is likely no one to tell you how to organize your orientees' information.

Communication Strategies

Although interoffice and postal mail are still options for communicating with others, email and phone calls are probably your most utilized communication strategies. Their ease of use, though, has contributed to a significant increase in the number of messages sent and received on a daily basis, and organizing all of these messages can be quite overwhelming. We want to offer you a few strategies to help you keep these messages organized.

Email

In today's healthcare world, email will most likely be the primary way you communicate with others. Because of this, you really want to keep your email messages organized. Having thousands of messages in your inbox will make it difficult to find emails easily and to stay organized. Additionally, most Information Technology (IT) departments have set a limit to the size your inbox can be...you will have to file those emails eventually! If you do it as messages come in, your life will be much easier.

Some email programs allow you to "flag" or "mark" the message as being high-priority or even automatically add it to a to-do list. This is a great way to get started. Some people will keep the message marked as "unread" if it's a high-priority email. Regardless of how you mark the important messages, once you have responded to or taken care of the request, you should move the message out of your inbox. You can move it to another folder if you want to keep it for later, but at least move it out of your inbox. You will be surprised at how much of a relief it can be to have an email inbox that can display all messages on one page, rather than having to scroll to find a message.

Probably the best advice for keeping your email messages organized is to create folders and subfolders for storing messages. Every person prefers a slightly different system, but Figure 8.1 demonstrates one option to consider. You could have a folder for every orientee or a folder for every cohort, or both. Additionally, in managing orientation activities, you probably want a folder for each class, activity, or committee in which you participate (see Figure 8.2). If you think a message fits into two categories, you could consider forwarding it to yourself (so that you have a total of two copies) and place one in each desired folder. Some email programs, such as Microsoft Outlook, will allow you to copy a message and place it in the additional folder.

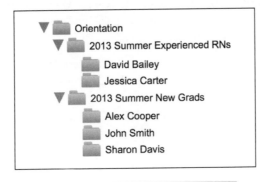

FIGURE 8.1

Methods for organizing orientees into folders and subfolders.

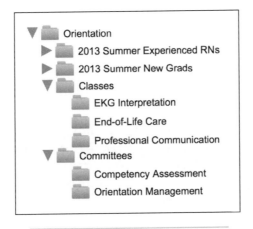

FIGURE 8.2

Methods for organizing orientation activities into folders and subfolders.

Some people prefer to skip meticulous folder management in favor of searching for messages based on a keyword. This can work too, unless the message happens not to contain the keyword you search. For example, if you were looking for all the confidentiality agreements from new hires during the past year, and you search for "confidentiality," you would not retrieve messages in which the new hire simply said,

"Here's my agreement." By having a folder devoted to confidentiality agreements, you would know where all of them were located. Given the amount of information most of us receive on a daily basis, we would not recommend the keyword approach. You will save yourself a lot of time and pain by using a folder system.

If you will not have access to email for several days (yes, you should still take vacations even if you are in charge of orientation), you would be wise to set up an automatic reply message that will inform the sender of when you expect to have access to email again and who he/she could contact if there is an immediate need. Also, before going on vacation, your email program may allow you to set up "Rules" that would forward certain emails to a special folder, so that your inbox does not become too unwieldy while you're gone. Rules in the email program can be useful any time, but particularly when you're away from the office.

Phone

Whether you have an office phone, a mobile phone, a pager, or even all three, this will be an important method for staying organized. Especially if you have a smartphone as your mobile phone, you can get additional information like emails, calendar appointments, and even to-do lists. Contact your IT department for assistance in setting this up.

Even if you don't have a smartphone, make sure your phone has a professional voicemail message for when you are unavailable to answer your phone. Additionally, if you go on an extended leave, set an out-of-office message with details of when you'll return to the office and who the caller can contact if he/she has an urgent need.

Managing a Calendar

Maintaining an accurate calendar is essential to staying organized. Whether it's meetings with administrators and new hires, teaching a class, or simply making time for lunch on a busy day, knowing where to be and when is key to meeting all your responsibilities. The simple part of maintaining a calendar is writing things down when you get invited to a meeting (or if details get changed). The more complex part starts when you begin scheduling the details of a major task.

Plan Ahead!

Although calendars can be useful to help you organize your day as soon as you get into the office, the real time management benefit will be seen in planning ahead...days, weeks, and even months ahead! Let's take the practical example of sending a new hire through orientation and onboarding. When a new person starts, you want to place every possible meeting on the calendar, and then reschedule if needed. If it doesn't make it to the calendar in advance, it may never make it.

Table 8.1 has a timeline of potential activities and meetings to place in your calendar when a new employee starts. As soon as you discover a new employee is starting, we recommend placing all of these events on your calendar in one sitting to make sure you don't leave anything out. However, you may have to wait until you have more details about the orientee's unit-level schedule before planning exact times. If you don't have all the details at the beginning, you could consider placing timed reminders or to-do items at the beginning of the week to provide you with a cue to confirm an appropriate time.

TABLE 8.1 *Activities to Place in Calendar When a New Employee Starts*

Background: You are the unit-based educator in a medical-surgical unit where orientation typically lasts 8 weeks, and the centralized educators are responsible for scheduling general hospital and nursing orientation. Your manager has just informed you that a new nurse will be starting 4 weeks from now.

TIME	ACTIVITY
4 Weeks Pre-Hire	Place new hire's start date on your calendar.
2 Weeks Pre-Hire	Schedule phone call (~15 min.) to talk with orientee and gather more information.
Week 1	Meet face-to-face with new employee during central orientation (consider scheduling a lunch meeting that includes managers and preceptors).
	Schedule at least 1 hour to provide new employee with a tour of the unit and other activities needed before taking care of patients.
Week 2/3	Schedule at least 15 minutes to simply check on the orientee and preceptor.

continues

TABLE 8.1 *Continued*

TIME	ACTIVITY
Week 4	Schedule meeting with manager, preceptor, and orientee to formally evaluate mid-orientation progress.
Week 5/6	Schedule at least 15 minutes to simply check on the orientee and preceptor.
Week 7/8	Mark orientee's tentative last day.
	Schedule meeting with manager, preceptor, and orientee to formally evaluate orientation progress and determine readiness for practicing independently.
Immediately Post-Orientation	Schedule at least 15 minutes on several days to check on independent orientee.
90 Days Post-Hire	Place a "Probationary Evaluation Due" item on calendar.

Obviously, this is just a rough sketch, and you are encouraged to meet with the new employee more frequently than this table recommends. Hopefully you can see how complex a calendar might become if you have multiple new hires in orientation at the same time. By placing all significant dates on your calendar as soon as you can predict them, you are more likely to stay on track. These frequent meetings with the new employee will also demonstrate to him/her that you care about his/her performance.

Paper vs. Electronic

Some people prefer paper calendars rather than electronic versions. But in today's healthcare environment, an electronic calendar is almost a necessity. Some people like to have both available (for example, the electronic calendar is for work and the paper calendar is for family), but be careful when adding events because you don't want to double-book yourself. In many electronic calendars, you can mark appointments as confidential or private so that others cannot see your personal appointments. You also have the ability to apply different color schemes to different types of appointments, so you can easily see what is a work-related meeting versus what is your kid's soccer game. Consider syncing your calendar with your smartphone or other portable device. Because most people always have their phones with them, a paper calendar will be one less thing to remember to have on hand.

Other benefits of having an electronic version of your calendar include:

- Accessible anywhere with a network connection
- Others can view or modify your calendar if they have permission to do so
- Invitations from others can easily be added to your calendar
- Frequent changes will not result in a "messy" look
- Easier to set up meetings with others who also have an electronic calendar
- Search function typically available
- Forward calendar events and invitations to others who need to attend
- Can add repetitive events (such as weekly or monthly meetings) quickly

Even though we recommend going paperless to stay organized, there is still benefit in having paper (or sticky notes) available. You will find something that works for you, but until then, try experimenting with different methods.

Ongoing Review of Orientation/Onboarding Program

We've mentioned the use of the ADDIE model throughout this book. Because this is a cycle intended to be repeated (and because the needs of the organization change regularly), you should set aside time for regular review of various aspects of your orientation and onboarding program. You should schedule these reviews far in advance for a couple reasons:

1. Ensuring the presence of key stakeholders for high-level program analysis and evaluation
2. Maintaining up-to-date learning activities

For the high-level program analysis and evaluation, you may want to consider scheduling a standing annual meeting with key stakeholders. By scheduling a meeting far in advance (up to a year), you can increase your chances that all the desired people will be there. From the perspective of current learning activities, you could schedule annual reviews of classes and modules by subject matter experts. Some organizations change so frequently that learning activities (especially those without a facilitator) may quickly become outdated, and you want to be certain new employees are receiving a relevant learning experience.

You also may want to set aside an hour each quarter to check for regulatory or other changes that impact your onboarding and orientation program. In addition to the annual review with key stakeholders, this will help ensure that your program stays up-to-date… and legal!

Computer Folders

For your dedicated work computer, you may want to place shortcuts on the desktop that link to your most commonly used folders and files. Especially when accessing files that are stored in subfolders of a shared/network drive, you can waste a lot of time searching for files. So, instead of clicking through multiple folders to get to your destination, place a hyperlink or shortcut in an easily accessible location. This could be on your desktop, or you could have a spreadsheet or text document that has embedded hyperlinks to desired files.

Once you've been managing orientation and onboarding projects for a few months, you will probably have several files on your computer that you are particularly fond of and have spent a lot of time perfecting. The last thing you want is for your hard drive to go bad and lose this information. Consider the following methods for having an extra copy available for a rainy day:

- Email a copy of the file to yourself
- Store a copy on a thumb drive or external hard drive
- Create a backup folder in a "cloud" or on your organization's server
- Regularly back up your local hard drive

Spreadsheets

Whether you're responsible for 5 employees or 500, maintaining an organized, easily searchable record of all relevant dates for orientation and competencies is an essential role of the educator and/ or manager. Most people will use some sort of spreadsheet to organize this information because you can search the spreadsheet for desired information and organize the information into reports, and because data input is relatively simple. Some organizations will create databases instead of keeping all information in spreadsheets, but database creation and management is a complex project that is beyond the scope of most nursing professional development specialists.

This section is not intended to replace the "Help" function in your software but rather to point you in the direction of some features specific to the role of a professional development specialist. If you're using Microsoft Excel and want a few extra tips, Alvin recommends *101 Excel 2013 Tips, Tricks & Timesavers* by John Walkenbach (John Wiley & Sons, 2013).

Our recommendations for designing effective spreadsheets can be found in Table 8.2. Several of these recommendations are represented in Figures 8.3, 8.4, and 8.5.

TABLE 8.2 *Spreadsheet Recommendations*

RECOMMENDATION	RATIONALE
Place only one word or date in each column (e.g., have a column for "First Name" and "Last Name" rather than just "Name")	This allows for filtering based on specific criteria and prevents inconsistencies in data input.
Use "Comments" for adding qualitative data	Most additional qualitative information is unique to that entry, so a separate column isn't necessary.
Consider placing a unique identifier (e.g., employee ID) in the far-left column	Facilitates integration of spreadsheet data into a database should that be necessary in the future. Also necessary for "VLOOKUP" formulas, if desired.
Add color to spreadsheet	Color makes the spreadsheet easier to read.

continues

TABLE 8.2 *Continued*

RECOMMENDATION	RATIONALE
Create a copy of the spreadsheet every year (e.g., "Education Spreadsheet 2012")	Keeps data succinct, as more education requirements are added or changed each year. Prevents loss of all data in the event of file corruption.
Add an "AutoFilter" toward the top of the spreadsheet	Provides easy ability to sort by items such as name, date completed, or even missing data.
Divide spreadsheet or workbook into smaller worksheets that are functional (e.g., by cohort or discipline)	Having a functional organization to a spreadsheet can assist with rapid retrieval of desired information.

Figure 8.3 is an example of a basic spreadsheet where we have listed all of the employees' names along with significant dates. Although we have only listed hire date, orientation completion date, and a few educational requirements, you could place any and all relevant dates into a spreadsheet. The second row (immediately under the heading row) is a blank row with a filter added. These filters (displayed by arrows) allow you to sort the data in various ways (for example, placing the information in ascending order by hire date to determine who has the most tenure). In the example listed here, the data is filtered and sorted by last name, so that employees are easily listed in alphabetical order.

	B	C	D	E	F	G
1	Last Name	First Name	Hire Date	Completed Orientation	CPR Expiration	Glucose Meter
2						
3	Brodeur	Susan	7/29/08	9/30/08	11/29/13	7/28/13
4	Clark	Dena	6/8/90	8/8/90	2/21/14	7/26/13
5	France	Debra	10/13/96	12/10/96	9/23/14	7/25/13
6	Jarvis	David	11/9/88	1/9/89	11/7/13	7/27/13
7	Jeffery	Bill	8/11/99	10/11/99	2/3/14	7/14/13
8	Mueller	Beth	1/4/08	3/1/08	8/7/13	7/23/13
9	Rutschilling	Jamey	5/13/12	7/13/12	2/25/13	7/9/13

FIGURE 8.3

Example spreadsheet.

Figure 8.4 has the same information as Figure 8.3 but with the addition of a unique employee identifier. Placing this column on the far left is recommended if you hope to integrate the information into a database (or intend on using a VLOOKUP function). The other addition to this figure is the presence of a comment. After a comment is added to a cell, if you move your mouse over the cell, a pop-up box will appear with the contents of the comment (in this case, the comment box states "Did not start with the rest of her cohort.").

	A	B	C	D	E
1	Employee ID	Last Name	First Name	Hire Date	Completed Orienta
2					
3	38729	Brodeur	Susan	7/29/08	Author:
4	24372	Clark	Dena	6/8/90	Did not start with the
5	65983	France	Debra	10/13/96	rest of her cohort.

FIGURE 8.4

Use of unique identifier and comments.

Figure 8.5 illustrates the creation of several worksheets (tabs). Each of these tabs, once clicked, will display a different worksheet within the same workbook (file). The three tabs on the left of this figure demonstrate the organization of new employee cohorts based on their hire date, and the three tabs on the right are organized based on discipline/profession of the new hires.

| Jul 2013 | Sept 2013 | Nov 2013 | RNs | UAPs | RTs | + |

FIGURE 8.5

Use of worksheets (tabs).

Learning Management System (LMS)

If you work in a large organization and have a centralized training and development department (T&D), this department may have purchased a learning management system (LMS). The department should be delighted if you approach them and want to track your orientees' progress on the LMS. You will want to work with the T&D folks to set up the classes and experiences in a way that makes it easy for you to track and is consistent with the structure the T&D department uses. This makes tracking and reporting a whole lot easier.

If you don't have an LMS in your organization, you may want to consider getting one. Even with an initial start-up cost, you may quickly begin saving money if your time is devoted to teaching as opposed to tracking. Many companies specialize in LMS development, and you could contact one of their representatives or search for information online if you want more information about what they are able to offer. Some questions you want to ask before purchasing a new LMS may include:

- Can we design courses to be housed in the LMS, or is it simply for tracking purposes?

- What are options for data input and data output (for example, manual and automatic)?

- Can reports be customized?

- Is there a one-time cost or an annual fee (or both)?

- How much do updates and improvements cost?

- Does the system integrate with other systems, such as performance management?

- What kind of technical assistance and training is available?

LEARNING MANAGEMENT SYSTEMS

If you do not have a centralized Training and Development (T&D) department, and if you have the budget, you might consider getting a Learning Management System (LMS) for your unit. Many of the LMSs are now available in the "cloud," so it doesn't take a lot of internal IT support. That said, you still need to work with your IT group to implement any type of LMS.

You will not want an open-source system, as it may be difficult to protect the confidentiality of your participants and their results. Here are some LMSs that might meet your needs. Please note that these are not recommendations but rather a partial list to get started in exploring LMS!

- *Saba—http://www.saba.com/us*
- *Success Factors—http://www.successfactors.com/*
- *Traincaster—http://www.traincaster.com/index.html*
- *Blackboard—http://www.blackboard.com/Platforms.aspx*

Paper Documentation

Some of you may not have all the technology available to you that we have discussed in this chapter. That's fine; we have ideas to help you, too! There are ways to organize your paper documentation as well.

- If you have orientees in a cohort, you should consider keeping all their paper documentation in a notebook marked with the start date. You should then keep their documentation by type (such as confidentiality agreements) in alphabetical order.

- If you don't have cohorts, keep paper files on each new hire, and keep those in alphabetical order. On the orientee's file folder label, you might note hire date. This can help you easily access your files when someone asks to see information on people hired on a certain date.

- You might decide to organize by type of training or documentation. If you do that, we would recommend that you use subcategories by date and then alphabetize by last name.

Records Retention

Your organization may have some policies or guidelines about records retention. Just as you should keep your tax returns for at least 7 years, there are guidelines about how long you need to keep certain types of records (paper and electronic). Please check with the records retention person to find out what you need to keep and for how long. Chapter 7 also briefly talks about this topic.

Building and Maintaining a Budget

Building and maintaining a budget will demonstrate to management that you understand money doesn't grow on trees and that you are willing to be objective in the distribution (and potentially the evaluation) of funds. You may not get all the money that you want (few people do), but by outlining the items you deem important along with their cost, you have an objective product to help facilitate discussions. The final approval will be in the hands of the manager, but as the subject matter expert, you are the best person to know what to ask for. Consider placing the following items in your budget:

- Orientee salary (although this is typically already included in organizational budgets)
- Teaching materials (books, office supplies, patient care equipment, software)
- Laptop and projector
- Camera
- Patient simulator and/or manikin
- Professional development materials (such as buying books or attending a conference for your development)

Conclusion

We don't expect that you implement everything as we have it here, but we hope you've learned a couple tips or gained a few ideas for getting (or staying) organized. Many of these skills and techniques are not something you would learn in nursing school or even during the orientation period to a new leadership role. Unfortunately, these are also the skills that can make your role very frustrating if you don't acquire them. In addition to what we have listed here, don't be afraid to perform a web engine search for complicated tasks or frustrating software error messages. Alvin learned to troubleshoot most spreadsheet errors through a web engine search of the error. Chances are high that you if are encountering a problem with some software, someone else has encountered the same problem and has posted a solution on the Internet. We're not saying that tackling all these organizational strategies or technology challenges will be accomplished overnight, but you can achieve a healthy level of organization that will help you keep your sanity. Good luck!

Questions for Reflection/Discussion

1. What tools do I have to stay organized?

2. Based on what I need to track, what tools make the most sense for me to use?

3. Does my record-keeping align with our organization's record retention policies?

KEY TAKEAWAYS

- *Keeping your work-related tasks and responsibilities organized is invaluable in performing your job duties, as it will save you much-needed time and energy.*

- *Even if orientation is your primary responsibility, all nurse leaders will be charged with managing large amounts of information and other smaller tasks (for example, budgets). Staying organized is the key to making sure everything is accomplished.*

- *There are many ways to stay organized, so don't be afraid to try something different or talk to others who have a "best practice."*

- *Many resources exist to help you navigate software and applications, so explore these and don't give up!*

APPENDIX

Essential Orientation Materials for Your Office

You may or may not have a physical office space, but regardless of where you manage your orientation activities, we would like to recommend a few resources for you to keep on hand. We would like to disclose that we have no personal or financial benefit in recommending these particular resources—they're simply what we use and enjoy.

Books

- This book, the *Staff Educator's Guide to Clinical Orientation* (obviously!): It will get you up and running while hopefully providing you with a concise overview of all activities related to orientation and onboarding.

- *Mastering Precepting: A Nurse's Handbook for Success* (Beth Ulrich, 2012, Sigma Theta Tau International): Preceptors spend more time with orientees than any other stakeholder, so their contributions are invaluable. This book will guide you and them on the path to excellent precepting.

- *The Ultimate Guide to Competency Assessment in Health Care* (Donna Wright, 2005, Creative Healthcare Management): Although Wright's book has a large focus on ongoing competency assessment, many of her principles apply to initial competency assessment, too. She takes a very different approach to this difficult task by making the process extremely practical.

- *Nursing Professional Development: Scope and Standards of Practice* (2010, American Nurses Association): This is a must-have for all nursing professional development specialists. Just like any other nursing specialty, nursing professional development has a scope and standards of practice. This text is the authoritative source of that information.

- *The New Mager Six-Pack* (Robert Mager, 1997, Center for Effective Performance): Mager is the grandfather of modern instructional design. Although the six-pack might seem like overkill at first, this is a great go-to series of books for anyone who is serious about being a great adult educator and designer.

- *The Accelerated Learning Fieldbook: Making the Instructional Process Fast, Flexible, and Fun* (Lou Russell, 1999, Pfeiffer): Russell's book will help you design and develop training more quickly, without sacrificing the rigor. Her book includes a CD-ROM with worksheets, etc.

- *Great Webinars: How to Create Interactive Learning that is Captivating, Informative, and Fun* (Cynthia Clay, 2012, Pfeiffer): Clay teaches seminars based on her book and really helps bring webinars to life. She shows the reader how to with great, practical examples. She reminds us to keep the learners front and center as we build webinars.

- *Creative New Employee Orientation Programs: Best Practices, Creative Ideas, and Activities for Energizing Your Orientation Program* (Doris M. Sims, 2002, McGraw-Hill): The author provides best practices and lots and lots of checklists for your use. Her approach is focused more at the organizational level, but many of the checklists could be adapted for use at a unit level. This one is an oldie, but a goodie!

Websites

- http://www.thiagi.com: Dr. Sivasailam Thiagarajan (Thiagi) started his business almost 40 years ago and his mission remains the same: "To help people achieve more through performance-based training that is motivating and effective." Thiagi is a great resource for games and other low-tech approaches to help groups learn information quickly and in a fun environment. He has many free downloads available on his site.

- http://www.trainerswarehouse.com: Trainers Warehouse provides items that you can use for (primarily) classroom-based activities. Want to set up your own version of *Jeopardy!* to facilitate learning a certain topic? Trainers Warehouse can help. Have a long classroom session and want some basic toys on the table to keep your adult learners occupied? They've got that kind of stuff, too!

- http://www.instructionaldesigncentral.com: Instructional Design Central is a website that provides resources and information for instructional designers.

- Stay up to date with your nursing journals and websites as well, and look for websites that focus specifically on being a professional development specialist in nursing! Here are some websites to get you started:

  - http://www.anpd.org: Association for Nursing Professional Development

  - http://pneg.org/: Professional Nurse Educators Group

  - http://journals.lww.com/jnsdonline: *Journal for Nurses in Professional Development*

  - http://www.nursecredentialing.org/NursingProfessionalDevelopment: Certification resources

1-Minute Literature Review

Even though books are great resources for developing or enhancing onboarding programs, there is also merit in having peer-reviewed articles available. Especially in organizations that have a large emphasis on evidence-based decision-making, you may be asked for "proof" that a particular change is warranted. Therefore, we want to provide you with several articles we believe are beneficial for you to have on hand. Due to the rapid nature with which new articles are published, this list may quickly become dated, but if you're short on time, this is a good place to start.

General Orientation/Onboarding Literature

Title: The Effectiveness of an Organizational-Level Orientation Training Program in Socialization of New Hires

Year/Author: 2000; Howard J. Klein & Natasha A. Weaver

Journal/Volume/Issue/Page: *Personnel Psychology*, 53(1), 47–66

Description: The authors look at the impact of organizational-level orientation in over 100 employees in different disciplines and industries before and at the 1- and 2-month marks. They found that employees who participated in an organizational-level orientation were more likely to be socialized about the goals and mission of the organization, as well as its history and people.

Title: Onboarding New Employees: Maximizing Success

Year/Author: 2010; Talya N. Bauer

Journal/Volume/Issue/Page: *SHRM Foundation Effective Practice Guideline Series*, 1–54

Description: Bauer addresses different (effective) approaches for onboarding new employees. She also explores short- and long-term outcomes that should be part of an effective onboarding program. Her Four C model is included in Chapter 2 of this book.

Title: New-Hire Onboarding: Common Mistakes to Avoid

Year/Author: 2013; Alexia Vernon

Journal/Volume/Issue/Page: *T&D*, 66(9), 32–33

Description: This short article addresses five key mistakes to avoid when onboarding, especially when onboarding new college graduates. The author discusses strategies for avoiding these common mistakes, as well as the importance of engaging your new employees on day one.

Nursing-Specific Literature

Title: A Magnetic Strategy for New Graduate Nurses

Year/Author: 2007; Diana Halfer

Journal/Volume/Issue/Page: *Nursing Economic$, 25*(1), 6–11

Description: This article describes one hospital's major overhaul of its orientation program, which reduced new graduate RN turnover from 29.5% to 12.3%. The hospital developed a holistic orientation/onboarding program that involved classroom training (general and specialty content along with advanced life support), structured mentorship, preceptor development, professional transition support, and debriefings.

Title: Specialized New Graduate RN Pediatric Orientation: A Strategy for Nursing Retention and Its Financial Impact

Year/Author: 2013; M. Isabel Friedman, Margaret M. Delaney, Kathleen Schmidt, Carolyn Quinn, & Irene Macyk

Journal/Volume/Issue/Page: *Nursing Economic$, 31*(4), 162–170

Description: In addition to demonstrating the financial impact of a well-developed onboarding program, this article contains several tables with content and timeline details of a yearlong fellowship program for new graduate RNs entering specialty fields (critical care, emergency department, and hematology/oncology).

Title: Orientation to Emergency Nursing: Perceptions of New Graduate Nurses

Year/Author: 2010; Barbara Patterson, Elizabeth W. Bayley, Krista Burnell, & Jan Rhoads

Journal/Volume/Issue/Page: *Journal of Emergency Nursing, 36*(3), 203–211

Description: This research study used qualitative and quantitative methods to discover strengths as well as improvement opportunities for a 6-month fellowship program for new graduate RNs working in an emergency department. Strengths included length of program, support from key stakeholders, interpersonal relationship development within cohort, and variety of learning materials and classes. Opportunities for improvement included dispersing class sessions throughout program (rather than at the beginning), focusing classroom content on specialty, increasing the use of simulation (and other interactive activities), and providing more debriefing and discussion opportunities.

Title: Solving the Retention Puzzle: Let's Begin with Nursing Orientation

Year/Author: 2012; Betsy Brakovich & Elizabeth Bonham

Journal/Volume/Issue/Page: *Nurse Leader, 10*(5), 50–53, 61

Description: The authors of this article used the Casey-Fink Graduate Nurse Experience Survey to explore the perceptions of new graduate RNs during their third month of employment. They describe the perspective of four different cohorts in the areas of skill and procedure performance, confidence and stressors, role transition, confidence and critical-thinking skills, time management, role responsibility, communication, and support in the work environment. This article provides a summary of what many new graduate RNs are thinking at the 3-month mark.

Title: An Interdepartmental Team Approach to Develop, Implement, and Sustain an Oncology Nursing Orientation Program

Year/Author: 2011; Nancy Kuhrik, Linda Laub, Marilee Kuhrik, & Kathy Atwater

Journal/Volume/Issue/Page: *Oncology Nursing Forum, 38*(2), 115–118

Description: These authors provide the reader with specific outlines and objectives of their orientation schedule. Although the content is specific to oncology nursing, their format could be easily adapted to your individual needs.

Title: Progress Meetings: Facilitating Role Transition of the New Graduate Nurse

Year/Author: 2009; Marlene Goodwin-Esola, Maureen Deely, & Nancy Powell

Journal/Volume/Issue/Page: *The Journal of Continuing Education in Nursing, 40(9), 411–415*

Description: This article details a practical method for meeting regularly with new graduate RNs to assess their progress and help them transition into their new roles. By meeting regularly and consistently to assess competency development, the new nurse not only transitions more smoothly, but also develops stronger relationships with the managers and educators.

INDEX